To my Oscar

ADVENTURES BRINGING UP A SON WHO HAPPENS
TO HAVE DOWN SYNDROME

FOR
THE LOVE OF
OSCAR

SARAH ROBERTS

AD LIB

First published in 2022 by Ad Lib Publishers Ltd
15 Church Road
London, SW13 9HE

www.adlibpublishers.com

Text © 2020 Sarah Roberts

ISBN: 9781913543129
EBOOK: 9781913543877

A CIP catalogue record for this book is available from the British Library.

Every reasonable effort has been made to trace copyright-holders of material
reproduced in this book, but if any have been inadvertently overlooked the
publishers would be glad to hear from them.

Printed in the UK

10 9 8 7 6 5 4 3 2 1

CONTENTS

INTRODUCTION

I never envisioned when I first had my eldest son Oscar that I'd spend a great deal of my time in negotiations. And I'm talking about the times I've had to metaphorically talk him down from a cliff. Thankfully no cliffs have actually been involved (I mean, Oscar near a cliff edge would be a disaster waiting to happen, quite frankly). But if you'd told me I'd be doing UN peacekeeper-type negotiations with my boy back when I'd had him, well, I don't know if I'd have understood. Surely kids don't actually do these sorts of things?

The thing is, how could I have possibly known that with his diagnosis, there'd come this much trouble …

Take for example the time we were walking down the canal and he decided, completely out of the blue, to take a flying leap onto a nearby barge. He was only three at the time and his sense of danger … well, there was none! Thankfully he didn't fall in, but it was there that my husband Chris and I had to tempt him back on to dry land.

Then there was the time we found him on the flat roof of our first-floor extension (yep, you read that right, the actual roof). Having climbed through our top-floor-extension window, he proceeded to run around the circumference, shouting at the top of his voice, clearly chuffed with his efforts. Instead of heading out there ourselves, knowing if we did that he'd more than likely start running around even faster, I ran downstairs to grab a Fab lolly from the freezer and a bag of Haribo I'd had stashed in the cupboard and we managed to lure him back in with his choice.

Then there was the time he stuck his arm up the car exhaust pipe, managing to cake his entire face with thick black soot. This was after I'd told him in no uncertain terms not to touch his face and even pleaded with him not to do so, but of course there are times when negotiations just don't work, right?

And I'm not blaming the Down syndrome here. I'm well aware, having had two other children who don't have Down syndrome, that kids, regardless of anything else, can do some really bloody stupid things at times. But Oscar takes things to a different level, he really does.

I suppose I should commend Oscar for his sense of adventure. And I suppose the fact that he's determined and independent is a good thing, right? I listen to other parents talk about their children and how they never stray too far from their sides and I wonder why I ended up with three kids who invariably head off in completely different directions. And although all three of my kids love to explore, there are two of them that get a certain distance away, panic they're too far away from us and scurry back. But a certain someone else couldn't care less how far they wander. In fact, they're far too busy having a lovely time, keeping us on our toes and, yes, you've guessed it, that certain someone would be Oscar.

I'm not sure about you but even without three kids in tow, going through security at the airport makes me a little nervous. The mere fact you have to remember to take your mobile phone and iPad out of your bag, take your coat off and then time it so you walk through at the exact same time your belongings get to the end of the belt, for fear that someone in the line before you might pick up your bits … well, it stresses me out. Combine that with taking all your own stuff, plus your three kids, all their stuff, your husband *and* all his stuff – in those situations, you're basically screwed.

So picture the scene. I'm about to go through security at Geneva airport. Flo is in her baby carrier attached to me, both boys are strapped in side-by-side in the double buggy. I've put everything on the conveyor belt (did I mention they had to check the bottles of milk and baby food I was carrying for Flo, too?) and watch it slowly start to be screened. Only at this point, security ask me to take my baby out of the baby carrier *and* get the boys out of the buggy, collapse it as it's too wide for the screening machine and then all walk through the scanner. You can imagine my face at this point.

The boys, clearly thrilled at the prospect of getting out of the buggy, jump out and run through without a care in the world. Chris follows only for the machine to beep. (Of course it does. It beeps *every* time we go through airport security because *every* time it's his flippin' belt!) By this point I can see Oscar and Alfie in the distance, running amok and about to enter duty free.

Now, I mean this with the greatest of respect but Chris has always been a bit pants at doing more than one thing at a time or anything with any kind of urgency. While he was busy collecting his iPad, phone, keys, bag, belt etc., having whizzed through the screening, I was basically dragging the kids back to where we were standing. Flo, now out of her carrier, was equally delighted and having sat her on the floor (no judgement, please) was herself about to make a break for it. Thankfully I could wedge her between my feet (where else do you put a baby in these situations?).

'Stand there,' I say to the boys. They laugh excitedly and start to run away again. Obviously, my authoritative parenting voice working a treat in this instance. I drag them back. '*Stand there.*' I'm a little firmer this time. They do. Right, now to grab all our stuff. I turn round to check they're still there, Alfie's stood quietly watching Chris and me, but Oscar's gone. Panic.

'Where's Oscar?' Alfie stares at me like most two-and-three-quarter-year-olds would, with an 'Am I bothered?' look spread across his face

'*Where's Oscar?*' I shout, perhaps a little too frantically/dramatically/like I'm auditioning to be Liam Neeson in the next *Taken* movie, but I'm a parent and I can't see my kid. My kid that happens to have Down syndrome (DS) and couldn't care less, remember? I kinda get the raised anxiety level.

'*I don't know,*' Chris shouts back, probably not as loudly as I had done but at this point we're most definitely causing a scene (if we weren't before with our out-of-control kids and conveyor belt debacle).

I run through security, over to the duty-free shop, look right, look left. Nothing. He's not there. All I see are hundreds of people milling around, without a care in the world, but no little dude in a green T-shirt and red shorts.

I run back to security, the panic rising.

'*He's here,*' shout the men and women behind the security desks and screens. They're chuckling to themselves; they have a new friend. In the few seconds I'd turned my back, Oscar had crawled under the security desk and is now wandering around their little area, smiling, waving and saying, 'Hiya.' They all think it is hilarious. Chris even takes a photo but my heart is still pounding.

You see, the thing is, among the DS community, Oscar is what's known as a 'runner'. In talking to other parents of children with DS it's not uncommon and, contrary to popular belief, he's not just running for the sake of running. I believe his escapes are calculated, that in his head he knows exactly where he wants to go. If a door opens, he is through it, quicker than a flash. We were sat in my mum and dad's garden the other day and someone opened the gate. Quicker than the speed of light, Oscar was across the garden, squeezing his way under the arm of the person opening the gate, shielding himself behind someone else, hoping he'd go unnoticed. My dad says Oscar must sense the draught when a door is opened and he seizes every opportunity to make a break for it.

Chris and I have to be on our guard whenever we are out and about with Oscar. We were attending a party just a few weeks ago and a whole bunch of our friends were there. While we wanted to chat with our friends we also said to one another that one of us would always be on 'Oscar Watch' at any one time. This might sound a little dramatic but knowing his ability to escape and the fact that he has a tendency to be a little over-familiar sometimes (a polite way of saying he's been known to bite) we always like to keep one eye on him.

When we go anywhere new or somewhere we haven't been for a while, I always do a check of escape routes. That might sound crazy but I honestly have to do it. On the day of the party I had, discreetly, taken a look round the garden, checking there were no holes in fences or bushes, that gates weren't open, that he couldn't get through the garage, and then I did the same with the front door. I felt assured that there was no way he could make a break for it. Fast-forward a few hours and while it was my turn to be on Oscar Watch my attention moved away for a minute or so while I got Alfie a drink but it was long enough. Just like that, Oscar was gone. He'd been playing in the living room, happy as Larry, but the next thing I knew he wasn't there. I wasn't too worried to begin with. I suspected he had gone out into the back garden to find Chris. I walked into the garden, had a look round, scanning the crowd, but he wasn't there. Still not too fazed, I decided he'd probably followed some of the older kids upstairs as he'd watched them previously and I could tell he'd wanted to go with them even then. So off I went scanning the area as I went, up the stairs, opening all the bedroom and bathroom doors, calling his name … but he was nowhere to be seen.

Panic began to set in at this point. If he wasn't downstairs, he wasn't in the garden and now he wasn't upstairs, where was he? He's made it out the front I thought, but the door was shut, it was heavy and I surely would have heard it if he'd gone out. I ran down the stairs, out the front door, looked up the street, but he wasn't there either. He *must* be in the back garden I thought, I *must* have missed him. Maybe he was hiding in the garage, as he'd gone in there to have a look round earlier. I ran back inside, through the house, out into the back garden. At this point a couple of people had noticed the panic on my face and started searching, too.

I shouted to Chris that I couldn't find Oscar, and Chris's immediate reaction was to run out to the front of the house, while I checked upstairs again. Maybe he was in a cupboard or under the bed? Realising that he definitely wasn't at the party and must be out the front I raced outside, too, heart in my mouth, hot, panicked, willing us to find him …

… only to see Oscar being passed to Chris by a passer-by and his wife who'd been walking their dog. They said he must have walked out of the cul-de-sac and crossed a main road as they found him walking on the *other side* of the main road, 'talking' on his toy walkie-talkie. They didn't know which house he was from but saw the balloons outside our friend's house and assumed he must belong there. I burst into tears. Relieved, grateful, but mostly I was cross with myself that I'd let this happen. As it turned out, the man who found him was a police officer – no less than a detective inspector. How fortunate was that! And I cried a little more, not only because I was so grateful he'd been found before he got hurt or taken but mostly because I was so mortified I'd let him down, when I was supposed to have been watching him.

Oscar? He was absolutely fine. Completely and utterly unfazed. So here's the thing – if you're reading this book because you've just had a little one with Down syndrome and you're looking for a bit of hope – there *is* going to be some, I promise.

I was searching for that hope when I started writing when Oscar was still very small. I had been discussing life with Oscar with a couple of friends, when I suddenly blurted out that I'd quite like to start a blog. I'm the world's biggest procrastinator, so I did diddly-squat about it for ages, but then Oscar had to go back to hospital to have heart surgery. I remember being at my mum and dad's house just a few days before he was going in and saying to my mum that I had felt this sudden urge to start writing some things down. If she thought I sounded strange, she didn't say so at the time and so off I went into her dining room to start straight away. It was going to be my way of making sense of everything and that was particularly true with Oscar facing serious medical treatment. I was worrying myself to death so writing or typing on a page was an outlet for me. It was somewhere for me to share my deepest and darkest thoughts, without fear or judgement. And do you know what? It really helped.

I wrote and I wrote some more and, to this day, I've never really stopped. I posted my first blog online via my own private Facebook page in January 2014. Oscar had his surgery back in May 2013 but I'd squirrelled that piece of writing away in my documents file on my laptop to bring out at a later date. Instead, the first thing that went public was me talking about Oscar's birth, his diagnosis and everything I had thought and felt. And I was a bit nervous about how people might respond to it, but I realised fairly quickly that I shouldn't have been – the response was an outpouring of love from friends and family that affirmed the fact I'd done the right thing by sharing.

I was encouraged to set up a public page which I named 'Don't Be Sorry'. This was a nod to the paediatrician who had begun the news of Oscar's diagnosis back in July 2012 with the negative words, 'I'm sorry, but we suspect ...' and was also a message to all my new followers (who were growing in number by the day) that, whatever their views might be about Down syndrome and whatever they thought having Oscar in our lives might have meant for us, I wanted to show them that there's never been anything to be 'sorry' about. That, for me, was the rationale behind starting 'Don't Be

Sorry'. It was about education, I guess. Showing people that Oscar and others like him can lead pretty amazing lives with the right support and input in place. So that's what I did. I started my blog and social media accounts and over time it grew until I started work on this book.

I always said to myself that I would tell my truth in my writing. It's not everyone's story because there is no one-size-fits-all when it comes to parenting a child with DS. In fact, there's no one-size-fits-all with parenting, full stop.

So this is my account of becoming a parent. And that's to Oscar, Alfie and Flo. Yes, you're going to read about what it's like living with a child whose considered 'different', but all children are different. You'll read about the highs and the lows, because I vowed I'd tell the truth about how I felt then – when Oscar arrived – versus how I feel now, after a few years. It will get a little serious for a bit. But bear with me. Big deep breath. It does get better, I promise you ...

CHAPTER ONE

'There are moments that mark your life,
moments when you realise nothing will ever be
the same and time is divided into two parts.
Before this and after this.'
– JOHN HOBBES (DENZEL WASHINGTON),
FALLEN, 1998

'If only I knew then what I know now' – this is one of those cliched, annoying phrases that people say with equally annoying hindsight. Obviously, we all go through life learning little lessons along the way but the life lesson I learnt five years ago was probably the biggest known to woman (or little old me).

You see, the thing is that life then changed massively. Not for the worse if anything for the better; it's just it took me a while to figure it all out.

I was thirty-four, had had an easy pregnancy and was

the sort of girl who kinda used to sail through life with an air of things pretty much always going my way. Bad stuff doesn't happen to people like me – that kind of attitude. Yes – I was a bit of a knob. So when my little guy arrived and twenty minutes later we received the heartbreaking news that they suspected he had Down syndrome, then, just like that, it all sort of fell apart.

It was two in the morning, it was dark on the ward and, if I'm honest, the future right there in that moment looked bleak.

'I'm sorry, but we suspect your baby has Down syndrome. He's showing signs of hypotonia [he was floppy] and appears to have facial dysmorphia.' This last was the structure of the face. I couldn't believe it – he's bloody beautiful, I thought. Who was this woman who was saying these things about my newborn baby? She was the paediatrician who'd been called to his delivery when the medical team had concerns in the lead-up to the birth. I can still see as clear as day her arrival in our cubicle. She stood at the foot of the bed and her words rang in my ears. She was cold. She appeared to have no compassion and soon left us to it.

I remember looking across to the other side of the ward and seeing another couple with their new baby in their arms, staring at us in disbelief. They tried not to make eye contact. I guess we were like car-crash TV for the maternity ward. I looked at Chris. My husband. The man I'd so wanted everything to be perfect for. The man I'd wanted to give the perfect baby. Only I hadn't. And there he sat, shocked, bewildered, scared. I felt like my world, in that instant, was ruined, if I'm honest. Lying in that hospital bed, staring at Chris, willing him to tell me that everything would be OK. But he couldn't. Right at that moment, he didn't know if it'd be OK any more than I did. We were two rabbits stuck in the headlights, looking down at our baby, feeling that our world had been shattered.

I wish I'd had a crystal ball the night I gave birth to Oscar so that when they told me they suspected he had Down syndrome, I could have looked at the future me, writing this five years on, and see that life didn't end then and there, and that I'm not sad. If anything, my life is pretty wonderful most of the time. If only I could have seen what my son's life would be. What his diagnosis would mean for us as parents. And that – even though our family's life looks slightly different to the way I imagined it would be for us – it is all as it should be.

I want to go back all those years and tell that girl lying there in the hospital bed to replace the feelings of sadness and anger with different emotions. With hope. Hope for her baby's future. I'm ashamed to say that at that time I had a stereotypical view of how I thought an adult with DS looked, having just had a child with the condition. I peered into the future and in my ignorance I saw an image of a man in his forties, holding hands with his elderly mother (me), wearing trousers that were far too short for him and sporting a dodgy-looking haircut. A view of what kind of life that man would lead. An unfulfilling and depressing life. How very, *very* wrong could I be.

I'd met Chris on my thirtieth birthday. He was friends with my sister's boyfriend (now her husband). He wasn't technically invited to my birthday drinks but my sister's boyfriend had asked if I'd mind a couple of his mates coming along and I hadn't, so they did. We didn't get together until a few months later. He found me on Facebook and requested to add me as a friend (something he denies, claiming it was the other way around. I have the notification to show it wasn't) and then invited me to see Elton John at the O2. I knew from that point he was a keeper. I mean who doesn't love a bit of Elton? But I couldn't go and when he took another girl in my place, I knew I really liked him because I found myself calling him after the concert to suggest meeting up another time. We went to a pub for a few drinks the next night, snogged in the car park and the rest, as they say, is history.

Life back then was pretty lovely. Romantic dinners, weekends away. We moved in together after nine months, he proposed on the top of a mountain after fourteen months and we were married two and a half years after we met. It was all perfect, I guess. We chugged along just the way I imagined we would, too, and I was enjoying every moment of it. I fell pregnant and we told our families on Christmas Day. At our twenty-week scan, they told us we were expecting a boy and from that moment we named him Oscar.

There was no indication whatsoever that anything out of the ordinary was going on during the pregnancy. We'd had the combined blood test at twelve weeks – when they took bloods from me and recorded a measurement of the fluid taken from the back of the baby's neck. The results had come back marked as a low risk – and let me just pause to talk about that term, 'low risk'. I hate the word 'risk'. When you look up the word on Google, it says 'a situation involving exposure to danger'. Is that what they think of Oscar? A danger? Anyway, I'll come back to that phrase later. Let's just say that nothing was picked up in any of the scans I had. Not the DS or the two holes in his heart he was born with. I don't blame the hospital for not picking any of it up. I know these things happen and when you get your one-in-fifteen-thousand risk (I much prefer 'chance') of having a baby with DS, there has to be that one. I guess we were that one!

The pregnancy continued to go well. I used to be a professional dancer and at the time was teaching dance classes at a full-time stage school for young adults going onto work in the industry themselves. I worked until I was thirty-six weeks into the pregnancy, teaching for seven hours a day. I was fit, I was healthy, and I felt great. It wasn't until my forty-week check-up with the midwife that anything seemed out of the ordinary. I remember it like it was yesterday, hopping up on the bed in the surgery and her listening to the baby's heartbeat. I'd gotten to know Marlene over the last few months as she'd been particularly nice to me, so I made sure I had been booked in with her for all my check-ups. We'd been chatting non-stop as I lay there on the bed, when suddenly she became silent and still. Her face went serious for a second or two and she asked me what I was doing later that day. I hadn't much planned. It was the height of summer and Andy Murray was playing at Wimbledon so I had every intention of heading home, putting my feet up and watching the tennis on telly.

'I think perhaps it might be a good idea if you head up to the hospital to be put on the monitor,' said Marlene. 'I'm sure it's nothing to worry about but baby's heart rate is just a little slower than where I'd like it to be, so just to be on the safe side you best get checked over.'

To be perfectly honest with you, I wasn't at all worried at this point. If she'd have been panicking then of course I might have been, too, but she was always calm and there I was, blissfully unaware of the events that were about to unfold. I decided against calling Chris. I didn't want to alarm him unnecessarily and, besides, he was working a good hour from the hospital. I thought, I'll just head on up there on my own and if there are any problems, I'll give him a call. So that was what I did.

I sat in the triage area of the hospital on a monitor, on my own, for a few hours. The midwives were lovely and didn't seem unduly fazed by anything so neither was I, really. There were a few moments when I'd get suddenly a bit panicky and feel tears spring up into my eyes but mostly I was OK. It wasn't until sometime later that the doctor came round to see me. The doctor told me, 'Now, I'm almost certain that baby would probably be fine in there for another two weeks, but because the heart rate is just a little slower, I think we best induce you and get him out.'

Whether it was me being completely in denial or just not understanding what was going on, I genuinely didn't feel worried in the slightest. The only thing I felt was excitement that I was about to have my baby. It didn't even occur to me that anything might be up. I called Chris, they induced me and Chris himself didn't turn up until a couple of hours later (this man has no sense of urgency, plus I'd told him to go home and pick up my hospital bag and not to forget pants and toothbrush, etc.) and we waited. Nothing at all happened for some time. We were laughing and joking. Mostly about the lady in huge amounts of pain next to me who was literally screaming the place down. Yeah – I laugh when I get nervous. I bounced on my yoga ball a lot. Still nothing. Chris ate grapes, I read trashy mags and that whole induced birth thing really was looking like a non-event at this point.

It wasn't until after midnight, on Saturday, 7 July 2012, that the midwife, having already been in a few times to check on me, said she'd like to hook me up to the monitor just to check the baby's heart rate. I knew the drill by now. It took a little while for the monitor to find a trace and regulate. While it did, she turned to Chris and me and said, 'If that number, the heart rate, goes below a hundred, press that button,' and she pointed to a red alarm button behind my bed. Something about her words panicked me. Chris was faffing around and at this point was not really paying attention. It had all been fine up to now after all. But something this time made me sit up and watch the screen closely after the midwife left. One hundred, ninety-eight, ninety-four, eighty-six … seventy-two …

'Chris! Look, it's going down!'

'Don't panic.' Chris came over to look at the monitor a bit more closely. As he did, the numbers kept dropping. The last thing I remember is seeing Oscar's heart rate somewhere in the sixties and shouting to Chris to press the alarm. He did.

Blog comments

Hi, my friend pointed me in your direction. We have just had a CVS [chorionic villus sampling] test done and been told our little girl has Down syndrome. I'm heartbroken. I don't know whether I'm coming or going. I was wondering if you could tell me of your experience? I'm worried about my two other children (age five and eleven) and the effect it would have on them and their life. Also, what would happen to her if anything happened to us?? I'm so scared and sad. All I've done is cry and be angry. I don't know where to go or what to do, everything looks bleak. We are seeing the midwife tomorrow to talk. My partner is set in his mind he can't cope with her having Down and for us to have a termination. Part of me wishes we didn't know. They said I have time to think about things but my partner just wants it over with. Truth is I don't know. I just know I'm struggling with the concept of saying goodbye.

Anon

Dear Sarah, our son Joe is five months old. We were given our diagnosis antenatally and I lost count of the number of people who responded with 'I'm sorry' when I told them. I even got a card from a friend of the family that said:

'Thinking of you at this difficult time'. Isn't that what people say in condolence cards?!

Emily Folan

Hi, I just wanted to say wow, thank you, your Facebook page and website has actually stopped me crying. I'm thirty-six weeks' pregnant and was told four weeks ago that my baby had DS even though I was low-risk at screening. I've been through every emotion going. I feel numb and so scared about my baby's future. I'm going in on Friday (thirty-seven weeks) to have him due to a liver problem I have. We have been told he has no health problems whatsoever – clear heart, liver kidneys, etc. he even has the ridge bone in his nose (well, that's what they are saying, but they also said I was low-risk). I'm trying to be positive but I'm a mess right now and I have a five-year-old as well who turns six on Wednesday who is so excited to have a brother. I went into work today, too, to say goodbye, so there were lots of tears as people all know.

Pamela Fitzpatrick

CHAPTER TWO

'She stood in the storm, and when the wind did not blow her way, she adjusted her sails.'
– Elizabeth Edwards

The hour or two after Chris pressed the alarm button in the hospital is all a bit of a haze now. Oscar's heart rate was dropping and I remember the noise of the alarm and it going right through me.

I remember the look of panic on Chris' face as what felt like an army of healthcare professionals ran into my cubicle to assess the situation. I was told by my midwife afterwards that when the alarm on a maternity ward goes off anyone not otherwise engaged must attend. They all crowded round my bed, then whisked Chris away to put him in scrubs. They deduced pretty quickly that they needed to do a Caesarean but didn't realise initially just how quick they would need to do it. They kept checking Oscar's heart rate on the monitor. Momentarily, it went back up. They did an internal examination and for anyone whose had an internal before, you'll recall it's not the most pleasant of experiences and those of you who've had an internal at speed will know it's, well, let's just say, 'Slap me in bread and call me a sandwich!' *Crrrikey!*

I remember them deciding that they needed to get Oscar out. And by that they meant get him out *now*. I was turned on my side into the recovery position and I got the shakes. Shaking uncontrollably. The midwife said I'd gone into shock and that I should try to calm down. They said that I needed a general anaesthetic as there was no time to give me an epidural. And I remember when they told me that Chris wasn't allowed in the operating room – I started to cry. This was going to be the scariest, most horrific, most panicked moment of my life and I had to do it on my own. Without my Chris.

Chris often describes the moment I was whisked off down the corridor. Not only was he scared for the life of his unborn son, he was scared that he might end up losing me. The noise of the medics shouting instructions at one another, the team bustling out the room, pushing past him as they went. Watching them running alongside my bed, to see us turn the corner out of sight, the doors swinging backwards and forwards behind us. Silence. There he stood, in his scrubs, all alone.

I was asleep for the next bit, so there are obviously not going to be any 'It's a strange feeling when they take a baby out by C-section and you can feel all the pushing and pulling' moments. None of 'the pride on Chris' face when they lifted Oscar into his arms for the first time' moments either and there's definitely not going to be, 'How amazing it was when they first put Oscar on my chest' moments because, well, I didn't feel or see any of those things.

In fact, the next thing I remember is waking up crying hysterically. One thing I've learnt over the years with Oscar needing GAs – general anaesthetic – for various surgeries, is that if you were feeling a particular emotion before they put you to sleep, you'll wake up feeling the same. So if you've been relatively calm beforehand, you will be when you wake. If you've been crying or feeling panicked, naturally you're going to wake up exactly the same way. Who knew, hey?

Anyway, I woke crying and I can recall a nurse holding me and telling me that everything was going to be OK. I felt groggy and it was dark in the room (by this point it was around 1.30 a.m.) and there at the end of the bed stood Chris, beaming. Cradled in his arms was what looked like a bunch of towels, but on closer inspection, I realised it was a baby. Oscar. Through the tears, I asked Chris if everything was OK and I've never forgotten what he said: 'Everything's perfect.'

His words were poignant as, for a few brief moments, all really was perfect in our little world. We had our baby, he was safe, we were complete.

The next bit you know. The bit about the paediatrician coming in shortly after I was introduced to my little man. The bit about how 'sorry' she was. The potential diagnosis. The shock, the headlights ... the rabbits ...

In the hospital bed, after all that, I couldn't possibly see how life would be for us. I couldn't even begin to imagine. So I sobbed. With more sadness than I've ever felt in my entire life, I lost it. Uncontrollable, all encompassing, full-body, lose-your-breath type of sobs. For the record, in hindsight, I was crying for me. Not for Oscar. Initially, it was all about how this diagnosis and having him was going to affect me and my lovely life. How it would affect Chris and me. We hadn't signed up for this, I thought, and, in that moment, I so desperately wanted it to go back to just the two of us.

Oscar was in the neonatal intensive care unit (NICU) for ten days. He'd had a problem with his heart (more on that later), hyperthyroidism (overactive thyroid, a dilated tube into his kidney and he was struggling to feed. Not the best outcome but, my god, did our baby fight up there in NICU. They couldn't believe the progress he made so quickly, especially with a dodgy ticker. On the tenth day of his stay, the day the hospital confirmed he did indeed have DS (yes, it took them that long to get the blood tests back!) we took our Oscar home.

When I think back to those first few weeks, I experienced such a mixture of emotions: joy that our baby was OK for now and doing well, but with a sick feeling in the pit of my stomach that I just couldn't shake; grief: I talk about this a lot and I know that some people who have children with additional needs take huge offence. But finding out my baby had Down syndrome was like mourning the loss of a loved one. I'm sure there will be people out there saying that I've never experienced losing a child and I couldn't even begin to imagine that type of loss. But I have lost family members that were my everything and learning Oscar's diagnosis felt much the same. It was a pain that felt like my heart was breaking. I had wanted to run out of that hospital on a number of occasions throughout the ten days Oscar was in there. I wanted to run out of NICU, into the corridor, down the stairs, out the hospital and just keep on running. I wanted to run because I didn't want to face my new reality. But of course I didn't actually run. Because somewhere, in all the pain and hurt and anger and grief, was love. Love for my baby. And while it took some time for the grief to leave me – because I was grieving for the child I imagined I'd have – over time that grief did disappear.

Two days after we had brought Oscar home I remember receiving a cut-out from a newspaper from

Diane, a family friend. She'd folded it up and sent it in a 'Congratulations on your Baby Boy' card. I remember at the time resenting all the cards that lined my windowsill. I hadn't felt like there was much to celebrate at that point and the cards were a constant reminder of how it could have gone had this been a happy time for me. (There it was again – poor old 'me'.) But eager to read the article, clutching at any sort of hope or reassurance anyone could offer me, I sat down. Tears began streaming down my face as I read. It was written by a father of a two-year-old boy with DS. He wrote of how he felt the day his son was born – this article could not have been better timed.

It was Tom Bickerby, writing a letter to his younger self for *The Times*:

You weren't expecting it, and you think your life is over. Well, it's not, and I'm going to tell you why … you will wish for terrible things; you will pray for your newborn baby to die – not just once, but a thousand times. Go with it, don't judge yourself, and the storm will pass. Lean on the people who love you but don't listen too closely to what they say for now; nobody can really know how you're feeling, or how to make you feel better …

The first and most important thing to say is that you are going to love this child. I don't mean love in a qualified, fond sort of way (although even that may seem unimaginable). No, I mean really love: on an elemental, mountains-and-oceans scale. And it won't be an effort. It won't be 'in spite of' anything. It will overwhelm you.

The second thing to say is that the future is your enemy and the present is your friend. You will gain absolutely nothing from languishing in dread about what you think will be difficult in the years ahead. Nothing is as bad in the moment as it was in anticipation, and often it's not bad at all. In fact, nearly all of it is really good.

The third thing to say is that other people are idiots. God love 'em, they will say things you'll scarcely believe; well-meant, but often ignorant, thoughtless, tactless, and breezily prejudiced. You will hear again and again comments implying that every person with Down syndrome is the same – all of them happy, life-and-soul types; crazy dancers who love a cuddle. Take not the slightest shred of notice. People with Down syndrome differ as wildly from each other as people without Down syndrome do ...

So don't think your life has just taken a horrific wrong turn and diverged forever from the path you wanted to take. It's still the same path. Being Alex's father will involve all the same joys and challenges as parenting any other child, just at export-strength.

And where's the harm in that? Whose deathbed wish is to have lived a life of slightly lower intensity?

You won't believe me, but in many ways you are lucky. You're going to meet some amazing people. They aren't saints, they're just supreme examples of normal humanity who feel drawn to work with children like your baby.

You would never meet them were it not for Alex and they will inspire you. You will find your son to be a magnet for wonderful, devoted souls. It will be your privilege to know them, and profoundly beneficial to you to feel so much gratitude. Most people don't get to experience that.

Mind you, there are other characters whom you should give a wide berth. Like it or not, you've just been inducted into an exclusive club, but don't make the mistake of thinking you have to get on with every member. Some of them are miserable company. There is a subset of parents of children with additional needs who make it their life's calling to become dysfunctionally over-committed, driven servants of their children's condition, in a way that seems ultimately to have little to do with their kids' wellbeing and more to do with their own self-esteem. Sounds harsh, and may be unfair, but don't waste time on them.

Trust your instincts about whose company will

have a positive effect on you and your family, and leave the others to mix with each other ... cherry-pick the life-enhancing friendships for a while and let the others lie fallow until you're ready. In some cases you're going to need to help them get over this new feature of your life far more than they'll ever be equipped to help you ...

So dry your eyes. You will be a good father to this boy, have no fear. Set aside your own feelings of loss and lift your gaze. While your love for Alex is still gathering pace, use the time to notice how readily everyone else adores him. The nurses in hospital, your family, your friends, even some strangers; they all respond to him in a way you're right to envy – with unconditional, instinctive devotion.

But give it time. When your love for this boy comes on-stream in all its might, it will make you the happiest you've ever been.

It was a piece of writing that literally picked me up out of my hole. Of course I didn't really believe any of what Tom had said at this point. It helped a bit but I remember for quite some time afterwards feeling this deep sense of sadness, like my heart had literally broken.

Blog comments

We didn't find out until after Seren was born. I'm glad I didn't know as it meant that I was able to just enjoy a very longed-for pregnancy without a load of stress and worry. We found out when she was five days old. I cried, a lot. Every time I read something I cried, as everything you read always has the worst-case scenario and I had a newborn baby who was just lying there doing nothing (as they do). So I stopped reading anything. For nine months. And I just enjoyed getting to know my little girl. I only started finding out more about DS as I was due to go back to work and figured people would expect me to know something about it! Maybe I was trying to pretend it hadn't actually happened but it really helped that by that point I could see my daughter developing and her own little personality coming through, and it wasn't all about the DS. I haven't come across anyone else yet though who's taken this approach. Most people want to know everything immediately. So my advice to any new parent is to follow your own path, we are all very different but you will get there your own way eventually, however long it takes.

Annalee Morris

We didn't know Freddie had DS until he was born
and I'm glad I didn't know. I was so uneducated
so when I found out when he was twenty-four
hours old, god I cried and cried and cried a bit
more until there were no tears left. I told the
midwife I didn't want him and that he wasn't
mine. I felt like that for well over a week. He was
in neonatal for twelve days and some days I didn't
even go and see him but as soon he got home,
I realised he was just still a baby. A baby that
needed his mum and so I gave my head a shake
and started educating myself. I went to the local
charity connected with other mums and realised
this journey wasn't as scary as I first thought and
now, six months on, although the feelings are still
raw and I do feel quite emotional seeing pics of
him in neonatal, I wouldn't change him for the
world. He's just Freddie and that's all he will ever
be to us.

Victoria Phillips

I think we tell ourselves that the way we found
out was the best way for us, as again it's fear of
the unknown. This is what we coped with so we
condition ourselves to believe this was best. We
had a postnatal diagnosis with our first baby
nearly three years ago and, yes, I think the biggest

advantage is having your beautiful baby in your arms at the time of receiving diagnosis. Also, I had a lovely pregnancy and am grateful for that. However, there is so much to learn/digest and you are straight into medical appointments, therapies etc. on top of learning to be a new mam that, if you had time to learn, prepare, deal with diagnosis prenatally, it might take away that intensity in the early weeks when you are just exhausted anyway. I don't think there ever is an 'easier' way or time to receive the news but we all seem to manage just fine whatever way we find out. Reach out to someone that understands, because that's what makes a huge difference, meeting families that 'get it'. And even though it's not OK now, it will be OK and it will be much better than OK. Our little rascal is the sunshine in our lives, along with his new baby brother. It's been a very long time since DS was my first thought in the morning and last at night. We really wouldn't change a thing.

Ger Cottrell

We declined screening but the twelve-week scan was so concerning they legally had to tell us apparently. There was a very high risk of Edwards [syndrome] or Patau [syndrome] and we were so terrified we would lose him, we paid for a private

Harmony test. While we were relieved it was
'only DS' there was still a lot of processing to be
done, especially as we were then told he had really
serious heart issues. I had a very tearful pregnancy,
with much of it spent either crying and/or
researching. However, I think most, if not all, of
the grieving had been done by the time he arrived.
I saw a counsellor a few times, too. There was
no shock or sadness when he was born. Just pure
joy and love. At the time, I wished nothing had
been picked up at the scan and that I didn't know.
In hindsight I think it was probably good we did
know. Two years on, I know I am the luckiest
woman alive.

Eloise Gee

CHAPTER THREE

'Be sure to taste your words before you
spit them out.'

L ife now is actually pretty special, I rarely feel sad. Of
course every parent worries, but those dark few
weeks that rolled into months in the beginning, in
hindsight, were a very small part of this journey.

Yes, I went a little cuckoo, I cried most days and
for some bizarre reason, felt the urge to announce to
complete and utter strangers that Oscar had Down
syndrome, just so it was out there and not an elephant
in the room, but things got better, I promise. This is the
time I've chosen to talk about now. It may sound bleak
(our story will get a bit more upbeat soon) and if so,
that's because at that point, life was.

The day we left hospital we decided to call in to

the supermarket to pick something up for dinner. We stupidly walked in carrying Oscar, he was still in the car seat and we quickly realised things would be a lot easier if we actually brought the pram in, so Chris went back to get it. Spot the first-time parents! While I was waiting with Oscar, out of nowhere came a voice, 'Hi, I thought you must have had him.' My friend Catherine. She hadn't heard we'd had our baby yet and she didn't know *the* news. In these early months, as I mentioned, I felt compelled to blurt out 'This is Oscar, he has Down syndrome' almost straight away. I don't feel that need now but with Catherine, I just needed to tell her. I remember the feeling of panic rise in me. The feeling of dread at having to say it out loud to someone.

'Well, we've only just got out of intensive care, we were in for ten days, he has a hole in his heart, a problem with his thyroid, a potential problem with one of the tubes into his kidney *and* he has Down syndrome.'

There it was.

I'd said it. My eyes stinging. A lump had caught in my throat. What did I want her to say? I actually don't know. I can't even remember what she did say as a response. Probably something lovely if I know her, but Chris interrupted us and the awkwardness was broken. That was to be the first of many introductions of my little boy and one I will always remember.

The next day we met our neighbours at the end of

the driveway while taking Oscar on his first walk. They were obviously keen to have a look in the pram and I remember cringing, thinking, please don't look at him. Please don't judge us. Ridiculous now as, if anything, I spend my time wanting people to look at Oscar. When I take him anywhere, I can honestly say, hand on heart, there isn't one bit of me that feels ashamed of him. How very different from that first meeting with the neighbours. Again, I felt compelled to tell them, again that lump in the throat forms and I choke on my words.

My mum had asked me, 'What do you actually want people to say when you tell them? What would you have said to someone before you had Oscar?' And if the truth be told, I really don't know. She reminded me that in hospital a lady I'd met said, 'It doesn't matter, he's still your son, you'll love him all the same.' And I guess it is that kind of response I want. Positivity, people, positivity. That said, while I don't claim to be the next Shakespeare myself and admit there's been more than one occasion when I've definitely said something ridiculous, my goodness, people say some really stupid things about DS.

Two days after leaving hospital with Oscar, an acquaintance (I won't call them a friend) said, 'Perhaps it was something you did late in the pregnancy that led you to have a child with DS.' I didn't have the strength to turn round and set her straight at that point. And how different my reaction to this would be now. Do people really think it's something I did during my pregnancy? Did I eat too many raspberries? Wear my belt too tight? It's times like this, I wish people didn't open their mouths.

When Oscar was about five weeks old I had to take him to the doctor for the first time. He had a bit of a cold so I decided it was best to get him checked over. Admittedly, I had felt some apprehension going to the surgery, as I was still struggling with coming to terms with it all. I knew the doctor wouldn't have necessarily read his notes. He was quite an upbeat man and seemed friendly enough but when he looked up at the computer screen, he started to read out loud, 'Trisomy 21 [Down syndrome], ASD/VSD heart problems, hyperthyroidism ... Wow, this is a medical student's dream, isn't it?' My blood boiled. It might be a medical student's dream to come across all these issues, but that's my son you're talking about – that's what I wanted to say. He then proceeded to ask me if I'd known about the diagnosis before Oscar was born. When I said 'No,' he replied, 'Really? That's bizarre, it's usually picked up.' Again, did he really think this was helpful? It wasn't.

'Did you have the tests?' Numerous – and I mean numerous – people ask this question. Consultants, GPs, Joe Bloggs on the street. I actually have no issue with people asking. I have asked other parents of children with DS. What I take issue with is that, when I say that I did have the tests and that DS wasn't detected and we were even considered low-risk, they always say 'Really? How unusual.' This is just an annoying response. First of all, of all the parents of children with DS that I've met recently, I'd say the majority didn't actually know before the birth. Maybe that's because, of those that have detected Down syndrome early, around 90 per cent choose to abort. Sad but true. And while we're on the subject, it's also very inappropriate to ask what we would have done if it was picked up. It's a personal issue and none of us couldn't possibly know until we're in that situation. I know what I think I would have done. I also know for a fact that I wouldn't change Oscar for the world so why are we even having this conversation? And, yes, that doctor at that first surgery visit asked me if I would have kept him, had I known at my twelve-week scan. Seriously.

People say ridiculous things. I've come to realise that over the years. Some people are ignorant and rude but most people I think literally have no clue about Down syndrome, so sometimes it's a question of verbal diarrhoea; mouth engaged without really thinking about what they're saying. And, hey, I've been guilty of that many a time. I'm not sure if I'm super-sensitive to it in others or maybe I'm just more aware of what comes out these days, but I'm sure I said some things without understanding, particularly in those early weeks and months.

A few weeks after Oscar was born, while I was wallowing in my own self-pity, I remember sobbing in my mum's arms. I wasn't sobbing because of the worries I'd had initially. It wasn't about what the future held for Oscar and me. Nor was I worrying if Chris and I would be able to cope. It wasn't the 'Could we love him?' or the 'Poor, poor me, my life is over' stuff. It was none of that. It was because I felt guilt. Guilt over my innermost, deepest thoughts. Around that time a very well-known celebrity had lost their baby. She had died. And I, while the whole country mourned, was pleased. I was pleased someone else was experiencing the pain and loss I felt. I was pleased someone else was hurting like I was, as I didn't want to be the only one feeling pain. I couldn't believe I could possibly think that. But I did. And there I sat, engulfed in my mother's arms, sobbing uncontrollably for my unforgivable thoughts.

The major turning point for me came when Oscar was six weeks old. I found acceptance and a chance to get my relationship with Chris back on track. When we were told about Oscar's diagnosis, Chris had cried. He grieved for what appeared to be about half a day and then he was fine with it. How was he not more upset, though? How could he be worrying about the borders in the garden? He'd made me so mad. So when Oscar was six weeks, we decided to take a holiday and get away. The relief was immense. The escape was what I needed and it also gave us the time we both needed. Time for Chris to get to know his son. Time for me to breathe. We also had a lot of time to talk. We needed to find 'us' again, because somewhere between 7 July and now, we had lost us. We talked long and hard. We listened. We didn't interrupt. And it worked. We found each other and even though we're far from perfect (he still does the gardening at very inappropriate times) we decided then that we would do everything in our power to make Oscar the best he could possibly be. We were united on that. After that holiday I came home a different girl. Don't get me wrong, there have been lots of wobbles along the way but for the most part, there's true genuine happiness... And when people say stupid things, you gotta laugh ... right?

Blog comments

I was sat in a restaurant with my husband and son. He must have been about two. An elderly lady and gentleman were sat on the table next to us. Taylor kept poking his tongue out at the man and the man was doing the same. The lady (I use the term loosely) came back from the bar/toilet and raised her voice to her partner, saying, 'Stop

it. He's retarded, can't you see?' To this day it
makes my blood boil.

Kayleigh Parsons

When I was fourteen weeks pregnant and just
found out my daughter would have DS, I got,
'Why don't you just get rid of it 'cos it will be
people like me that will end up paying for it 'cos it
will be a burden on society.'

Jannine Hooper

Health visitor at baby clinic when I pointed out
his DS section in his red book: 'Oh! [Leans in and
whispers] Oh, well, he gets away with it, doesn't
he? I just thought his dad was Chinese.'

Sarah Ojar

One kind old lady helpfully suggested we moved
away from the nearby pylons to avoid having any
more of those.

Jenny Asbury

Another mother pointed to my son in the
playground and said to me, 'Oh, I had really high
risk for that. Thankfully, she [pointing to her
daughter] doesn't have it.'

Hannah Rajgopaul

My uncle said Lucus looked like he was growing out of his Down's! A different aunt said I caused his DS by having the flu jab!

Kellie Evans

A conversation between a hospital midwife and myself when Finn was less than a week old in hospital:
Midwife: 'He does not look like he has Down syndrome.'
Me: 'Yes, lots of people are saying that but he does.'
Midwife: 'We had a baby in here recently that really looked like he had Down syndrome.'
Me: 'Oh … OK … And – did he have Down syndrome?'
Midwife: 'No, but the parents were really ugly.'

Helen Jehu

CHAPTER FOUR

'HOPE – Hold On Pain Ends.'

W hen I first had Oscar, I also had a preconceived idea of what a family looked like with a child with Down syndrome. And, since having him, I've realised that the way I used to perceive Down syndrome is seemingly the way the large majority of the population view it, too. And I so get that. I really do. Because let's face it, the large majority of the population haven't lived it like I have. Why would they even begin to understand my reality?

I thought we'd always be sad. I thought we'd never laugh again. You know – the proper pit-of-your-stomach, real belly-laughs you do when you haven't a care in the world. It would take a long time to really do that again. If I did laugh, I'd often stop myself, catching my breath when I remembered how much it all hurt. Before Oscar was born, and after I stopped dancing professionally, I used to teach dance. I taught for various schools, both children and young adults, all of varying abilities. In one of those classes, which I took for just an hour a week, was a bunch of kids with Down syndrome. And all the while I would come out of that class, my heart bursting with love, admiration and pride for how brilliant these kids were. But when I fell pregnant with Oscar, I didn't imagine for one single second that I'd end up having one exactly like them. I'd expected everything to be perfect. Everything to be normal. And if I'm brutally honest, I didn't want a child like them. I didn't want Down syndrome.

Watching myself write this now, reflecting back, makes me squirm. Because although I knew these particular kids were amazing and I'd seen first hand that their families weren't sad and that they went on holiday (yes, that was one of my other warped impressions, that families who had a child with Down syndrome didn't have a break) and were leading full and happy lives, my main issue is that I didn't want 'different'. I didn't want our life to be anything other than normal.

In the weeks leading up to Oscar's birth, Chris and I had attended classes with the NCT (National Childbirth Trust). A group of us met every Wednesday evening to discuss our pregnancies, birth plans, what happens in labour, pain relief, looking after our newborns and tips for early parenting. I'd loved it. And I'd been really excited to get to know the girls in the group, mostly because when you first have a baby, these NCT classes and the 'new friends you'll make' seemed to be all everyone ever talked about. Aside from the fact that it was so insightful to hear what to expect, I also loved that we got to meet other couples going through the same experience at the same time as we were. We were all very different, of course, but I guess we all shared the same focus – our babies.

One thing I do recall about these classes is that they didn't really concentrate too much on when things didn't go to plan. I don't blame them, as I'm guessing the whole traumatic birth, the undesirable outcome angle, would probably freak a whole heap of women out. A whole heap of women that would have paid a whole heap of money to hear how great everything was going to be. But the class did bring up DS. And the fact that it would be an unexpected diagnosis. But it was brought up around about the same time they mentioned stillbirths, which to this day upsets me. Never having lost a baby myself but working on the assumption that giving birth to a baby who has died in the womb is the most unimaginable pain one could ever experience, I can't see how a postnatal diagnosis of DS falls under the same category. It's just beyond me. That being said, I have already talked of a grief of sorts, as the dream of my typical child slipped away. I guess in hindsight, the NCT class were trying to go with 'When life doesn't go the way you plan it to', which I sort of get. Sort of.

The NCT course leader read out a poem called 'Welcome to Holland', the premise of which was when you have a baby with DS, it's like landing in Holland when you were expecting to arrive in Italy. It talks about how you'd wanted to ride in a gondola in Venice. How you'd brought the guidebooks for the Colosseum but when you land, you're now actually in a completely different country. I suppose you would be pretty gutted if that actually happened, right? The poem harps on about Holland being slower-paced than Italy and less flashy, and I guess in parts it's a really rather poignant piece of writing. Perhaps it's even a comfort for some. But equally it was also pretty depressing as it highlighted how 'different' life was now going to be and, well, at that stage of the game, that's the main thing you're freaking out about.

The course leader finished the poem and we all shifted awkwardly in our seats. She asked us if we were all OK and if anyone wanted to add anything and I recall one of the girls referencing her uncle who had DS but I can't remember what she said in detail. All I remember is thinking, make this stop. Make her stop talking for the love of god. Let's move on to placenta delivery and being stitched up, none of this 'dreadful outcome' shit.

It made me feel uncomfortable. I'd felt uncomfortable listening to the poem, too. And just like that it was over and, in all honesty, I didn't give it another thought.

By that time we had had the screening for Down syndrome, which came with my twelve-week scan. I had the combined blood test and they'd taken the nuchal fold measurement from the back of the baby's neck. We had received a letter just a few days after the scan to say all was well and that our 'risk' of having a baby with DS was low at 1-in-350. You are deemed high 'risk' if your results come back as being 1-in-150 or lower. In hindsight, now I think about it, 1-in-350 to me doesn't sound that great. But as a friend once put it, if you had 350 cups on the table and on the bottom of one of those cups was a red dot, what are the chances of you actually picking out that one with the dot? It seems unlikely. The thing is, I have known some women who've had babies with DS after being told their 'risk' was one in ten thousand. They just turned out to be that one. I also know of others who were one-in-thirteen and didn't end up having a baby with DS. My point being that the screening doesn't really seem to be worth the paper it's written on. Unless any of those women had a more definitive test to determine whether that baby had Down syndrome (a test such as an amniocentesis or CVS – chorionic villus sampling) there is always a chance, whether it be low or high 'risk'.

Anyway, I digress … as it turned out the NCT girls

and the support at the time were a good thing. We swapped late night emails about sleep issues or how many ounces of milk our babies were taking and it was a welcome relief. Sitting around drinking coffee, while the babies slept on blankets on the floor, for a while there, helped immensely. But some days I felt like I was on a Waltzer ride at the fairground that I desperately wanted to get off. You see, being around the other mums and having a daily reminder that their circumstances had all worked out, at times, really, *really* hurt. Why had it been me? Why hadn't one of them had the baby with DS? I used to torture myself with these kind of internal musings for months.

Some of the women in the group were older than me. I'd felt cross that as one of the youngest, why had it been me? Wasn't it proven that older mums with dodgy eggs had babies with DS? It is true that researchers have found that it is more likely for an older mother to have reproductive cells with an extra copy of chromosome 21. So an older mother is more likely to have a baby with Down syndrome. However, most of the babies who have Down syndrome (about 75 per cent) are born to mothers who are thirty-five or younger. This is because older mothers tend to have fewer babies. Only about 9 per cent of total births occur in mothers over thirty-five, but about 25 per cent of babies with Down syndrome are born to women in this age group.

For their part, I'm sure some of the other mums in the NCT class felt awkward themselves, walking on eggshells around me and careful not to say anything to offend. But I'm so very aware that none of this was their fault. I put all of this on myself. All of my concerns were my own issues and it was going to take me some time to be OK with it all.

Looking back now, I think things were in fact easier in the early days, in a practical sense. Oscar was just a baby, doing things that most babies did. But as time went on and those first few months passed, it became apparent to me that Oscar was starting to lag behind. His first smiles were a little later, his head control nowhere near as strong as the other babies, he didn't roll over for a while, or sit up as soon and, with every text or email or photo of their babies, doing all those things, it reminded me that our baby wasn't. Of course now I know, having had two supposedly 'typically developing' children since Oscar (more on that later), that all babies, regardless of additional needs or not, do things at their own pace. But at the time it started to get to me. In much the same way that I found baby groups and classes really hard, I worried that people were looking at Oscar weirdly, wondering why he looked the way he did and panicking that someone might actually ask. In those days I was still very blurty (although I'm pretty sure that's not even a word). What I mean by that is that I'd have this uncontrollable urge to blurt out that he had DS, in case people looked at him and wondered. Of course, the reality was they probably didn't even really care.

Baby-sensory class was really hard for me. I'd wanted to sign us up to do it because I'd wanted us to be as normal as possible, only as soon as I had, I regretted it. I think Oscar was around seven months when we first started and I remember having to prop him up between my legs into a sitting position because he couldn't sit independently. All the other babies sat up beautifully but Oscar couldn't. I felt people's stares. I saw them looking sideways at him or doing a double-take when they saw that his face looked a bit different to that of their little one. Some people would smile warmly but most, I felt, wouldn't make eye contact and would instead look away. I used to think back then that these women weren't being very friendly because they didn't want to have any kind of association with us. They felt relieved that their babies didn't have the condition, silently thanking god that it was me, not them. But was that the truth? I'm pretty sure these women did all of the above because of *me* – I made them feel uncomfortable. So when I finally relaxed and was OK with Oscar's diagnosis myself, I realised everyone else appeared to be, too. I've since gone back to baby groups with each of my other two children and I've come to understand there are just some people out there who just aren't very friendly. Some women need to have a word with their face, to remind themselves that their lives are pretty frickin' lovely, if they're getting to sit in a baby sensory class wafting floaty scarves in front of their child's face.

Baby groups may have been hard in the beginning but one of the overriding emotions I felt back then, something that is hard for me to admit now, is that I spent an awful lot of time in the months that followed Oscar's birth hoping that someone else would have a baby with Down syndrome. Friends who were pregnant, friends of friends who were, too, family members or extended family members ... each time any one of them gave birth, I'd secretly wanted them to experience what I had. I didn't want to be the only one, you see. I had wanted others to feel what I had. And those feelings took some time to leave me.

The thing is, none of my friends, family or extended friends and family have given birth to a child with Down syndrome since. Because the reality is, it's highly unlikely that anyone would. I guess that's probably why I felt so gutted about it ... because if it was that unlikely, why had it been us? When I finally got over myself – and for the record here I appreciate I may sound like a self-absorbed twat to a lot of people reading this, for feeling the way I had until this point – slowly, slowly I started realising that a life with Oscar in it wasn't as bad as I'd first imagined.

A few months ago my best friend's mum passed away from Alzheimer's. She was young and it wasn't fair. Just last month my sister found out her husband had been cheating on her and, as I write this, another friend is battling cancer. While I'm not likening Down syndrome to these awful events, I am popping them all in the same category of life not going the way you plan it to. Because if there's one thing I've learnt in my thirty-nine years on this planet, it's that sometimes we find ourselves on a completely different path to the one we expected.

I hope it's OK to admit all the things I felt in the beginning. It's been hard for me to write them down, but important for me to document what was really happening for me, in case there's anyone else out there feeling the same way now. Equally, it is important to me that people understand where I was at in those early days. It was a process that I had to work through. And every morning, when I woke and opened my eyes, Oscar's diagnosis was the first thing I thought about to begin with, but over time I realised I didn't feel quite as sad as I had done the day before. And so it continued. And slowly the fog began to lift.

Blog comments

Hello! This may seem like a completely random message for you to get but I really wanted to contact you. My uncle is fifty and has Down syndrome. I could only have wished for him to be brought up in today's society with people like yourself for my grandparents to seek support from. Unfortunately, they were left feeling very isolated – luckily they are amazing people and despite the lack of support they received by *everyone*, treated my uncle like any other child, gave him all the opportunities they could and proved everything every medical professional and passer-by said wrong. He has turned out to be the most amazing, semi-independent, hilarious, courageous and all round good egg!

Laura Birch

Hi, I'm a PA for a twenty-five-year-old lady with DS. She is now part of our family, in the fact that both my partner and eleven-year-old son love to be around her as much as I do. K still lives with her parents and enjoys a full, active life … K and I have some fab times going to different sports activities, the theatre, the pub, which is all great for her, however – for my partner and son (and me) she has taught, tolerance, patience, a different way of communicating and for them to understand choice and difference! The point I want to make is Oscar will teach his peers and

their families the really important stuff about life
and that different ability doesn't affect your rights
to a happy life with choices!

Anon

CHAPTER FIVE

'If there is no struggle, there is no progress.'
– FREDERICK DOUGLASS, 1857, ON
WEST INDIAN EMANCIPATION

For the first few months, I was very up and down, one minute feeling so completely in love with my baby but the next so very low.

My mum remarked some time later that although I smiled throughout that time, she could see a real sadness in my eyes. When you think about Down syndrome, most people think about learning difficulties that come with that label. I had had no idea that there is a list of associated potential health problems. Now, don't get me wrong, I can name a whole load of children with Down syndrome who have no health concerns whatsoever but fairly quickly we realised that Oscar had a number of complications, which I'm certain contributed greatly to my feelings of sadness.

Oscar had spent ten days in NICU when he was born. Initially, he'd needed some oxygen. He'd had jaundice and needed a bit of extra help with feeding at first. By the way, if you're reading this and have just had a baby with DS yourself, there is a big bad myth about babies with DS being rubbish at feeding. Just to put your mind at ease, sometimes our little ones do find it harder but other times they're amazing and take to the boob with no problem at all. I think because some babies with DS may be weaker due to heart problems, they may tire easily and therefore not have such a strong suck. This may have been Oscar's problem, if I'm honest. They found that he had two holes in his heart (ventricular septal defect, or VSD, and atrioventricular septal defect, or AVSD) and even though they said that at this point they weren't too bad at all, he really struggled with feeding in the beginning. For the first few days he was tube-fed, with me trying to breast feed every few hours. I wanted to make sure I gave him my colostrum (the good bit, according to the lovely NICU nurse who was looking after us) so I gave boob-feeding a go. Although I was OK, I was by no means a natural and I mainly spent the large majority of my time pumping my breast milk in the NICU kitchen.

When Oscar had his heel prick test, something they

give all newborn babies here in the UK, the medical staff picked up that he had hypothyroidism and would therefore need to be on medication for the rest of his life. To monitor the thyroxin levels in his body, they'd need to do regular blood tests to make sure he didn't need a higher or lower dosage.

He also failed his hearing test in the beginning, so they re-tested him and he failed again. It turned out he had glue ear which isn't all that uncommon with DS but was the beginning of our ongoing battle with his ears, which I'll go into later on.

If you google 'Down syndrome' and 'health-related problems', you'll be met with a long old list. In fact, if I had one piece of advice for new parents dealing with a pre or postnatal diagnosis, it's to step away from the computer. DO NOT GOOGLE, whatever you do. You'll meet heart defects, hearing loss, vision problems, infections, hypothyroidism, blood disorders, hypotonia (poor muscle tone), problems with the upper part of the spine, disrupted sleep patterns and sleep disorders, gum disease and dental problems, epilepsy, digestive problems, coeliac disease, mental health and emotional problems – it's so depressing. And, yes, while all these can happen, equally they might not!

I read somewhere that a couple who were expecting a baby with DS were told by their consultant that if they chose to continue with their pregnancy (and, yes, sometimes when people find out they're expecting a baby with DS, healthcare professionals work on the assumption that they decide to terminate), that their baby would have a 42 per cent chance of developing cancer in their lifetime and 17 per cent chance of a stroke. They were then handed a leaflet of the many risk factors and told that they could be booked in for a termination the next morning.

This was at the twenty-week scan and, much like me, the couple felt that the tone and mood of the medical professionals around them was sombre. They chose not to abort but realised afterwards that the statistics they'd been given about the condition in question about DS were exactly the same as the average human risks for these diseases. That a person with DS was no more likely to get cancer or have a stroke than the next person. And while this couple didn't actually terminate, they could have done, on the assumption that their child was more at risk of developing these diseases.

You see the thing is, when people are dehumanised by being labelled, with a bunch of statistics or the name of a condition, they become that condition before they are anything else. It's almost impossible to form a balanced view because the other side – the positive side to having any child – is hard to put into words, let alone bullet points in a leaflet. So seriously, folks, don't google whatever you do.

As well as the health-related stuff, I remember feeling completely overwhelmed by the long list (another list) of the professionals that were to have input into Oscar's development – physiotherapy was the first service he accessed but others spoke of portage, speech and language therapy and occupational therapy, too. I mean, who even knew so much went into the development of a kid with Down syndrome? I certainly didn't. Didn't have a clue and it wasn't until I met with Oscar's community consultant paediatrician, when Oscar was five weeks, and her telling us that she'd refer us for this service or that intervention, that it all became a lot clearer.

Oh, and before I go on, I should mention Oscar's paediatrician, Dr Hill. This was a lady we'd met briefly at Oscar's bedside when he was in NICU (she wasn't the lady who said 'I'm sorry', by the way). She'd been really nice but we'd been introduced to her before Oscar's diagnosis was confirmed, when we were still waiting on the results of the blood test. I knew we'd been referred to her because she specialised in DS and, well, that fact got my back up. So much so that when she came back to meet us at the hospital a few days later, I said to Chris that I wasn't going to talk with her as 'Oscar hasn't officially been diagnosed and it may be that the hospital staff have got it all wrong' (yep, DENIAL). I basically went and hid in the cafe and ate cake. What a knob (me, not Dr Hill).

But Oscar's paediatrician turned out to be essential, pointing us in the direction of the services that were available. At that first appointment she referred him to physiotherapy and shortly after we were put in touch with physiotherapist Jane. She was there from the beginning to show us exercises – oh, wait, not exercises; we're not allowed to call them that are we, Jane? – or rather the 'fun games' we could play with our little one. These games were there to encourage children like Oscar to improve on their gross motor skills. When Oscar was first referred, he would always lie with his head to one side. He was floppy and had zero head control. We look back now and realise that, although babies with DS are known for their poor muscle tone, the fact that he had a weak heart can't have helped with his ability to progress. In short, he must have been knackered all the time.

Jane helped him with side-lying, lying on his tummy, from moving his head side to side, pushing up, sitting up, pulling up and, eventually, walking. I recall in the beginning how straight-talking she was and how on occasion I'd come away feeling deflated. I suppose she'd seen it all and wasn't going to sugarcoat anything for me.

'Oscar will need some special supportive boots for when he starts walking,' she said on one occasion. It made me cross and I thought to myself, actually do you know what, Jane? Maybe he won't! Maybe he'll walk super-early and without the need for some stupid supportive boots. Maybe he'll be the first baby in history to do everything super-fast and nobody would even notice the delays (there it is again, people: denial). But of course she knew best and the 'special' boots, I have to admit, once I'd finally gotten over myself and actually put them on him, worked.

I think I needed a kick up the butt at times. I'd been superficial, worrying that the 'special' boots would have made him look 'special'. So he wasn't wearing the Converse trainers I'd so wanted him to wear, he would in time, right? (To give those of you reading this a teeny bit of hope if your little one's not walking yet – he did!)

Jane came to our house every other week for the physiotherapy sessions and Oscar would have hydrotherapy in the pool every second Wednesday. The water was amazing. He loved his swimming and when I finally let the feelings go and finished with the 'Poor me, poor Oscar' pity-party I created about the fact that we now had to attend 'special' hydrotherapy classes, I saw the huge benefits to his core strength. You see, the first time I went to the pool with him, I'd felt really sad. You know those clips on *Children In Need* that make you all emotional, when you see the kiddies enjoying the new facilities that come from the money raised for charity? Well, yeah, I thought we looked like them. I felt like an extra on a *Children In Need* clip. There we were.

In the pool with children who had such a wide range of complications and needs and yet all I was thinking was, this wasn't what I'd signed up for. (Another one of my selfish 'Why me/us?' moments.) But, over time, the feelings passed. I realised the children in the pool were actually doing just fine. Some of them couldn't walk when they started, but they learnt how to and they came in with the biggest, beaming smiles. Smiles that said, 'Look at me! Look at what I've achieved!' So the sadness only lasted a little while and in the end, if anything, I felt happy. Happy seeing that, along with the others, my little boy was thriving. He loved the water and I didn't have to meet the extortionate fees that some of my friends were – and are – paying for swimming lessons. God bless the NHS for our bi-monthly *free* swimming classes, right?

Alongside the referrals that the community paediatrician made, I reached out around about this time to a local support group. Before I'd had Oscar, as I said, I had taught dance and drama to a handful of kiddies who happened to have DS and who were all members of the charity PSDS ('Providing Support for Children with Down Syndrome and Their Families'). It was quite ironic to think that I had been pregnant with Oscar and already been a part of such an amazing organization working with the condition.

And since then, the trustees and the charity have

become such a massive part of our lives. They've been instrumental in showing Chris and I that everything really will be OK. That just because you've had a child with DS, doesn't mean you won't go on to have more children, that you will still be able to go out to work and that life, actually, really is rather normal. I continued teaching for PSDS after I had Oscar and I remember, on my first session back having had him, being worried that I might feel weird about it all. It had always been something I'd loved and looked forward to every week, but after having Oscar, these classes were surely to have a big impact on the way I was feeling. How would I see them now? Would I look at these children differently? Would I fear for Oscar's future? On the contrary, if anything, it gave me hope. I saw that these children were smart and brilliant individuals and I can remember as clear as day the first time I taught them after I'd had him, I thought that if Oscar turned out to be half as amazing as these guys were, we were gonna be just fine.

PSDS held a weekly playgroup called Digbies. In the main hall, toys and games were set up for the babies and toddlers, mums and dads were served tea and coffee and could just hang out with other parents who just happened to have a child with DS, too. In the rooms off the main hall they had a speech therapist, an occupational therapist, a music therapist and a teacher, all of whom offered our children the different therapies, from an early age. It was incredible. Aside from all the therapies offered, which in itself gave us the knowledge and understanding of what we could be doing with our children, they offered the most amazing emotional support. Their mantra was that with early intervention, there is no limit to what our children can achieve.

I was nervous at first, thinking that I was going to find a room full of really sad and depressed people with vacant babies. How very wrong could I be? I remember driving home from Digbies that first week and feeling this huge sense of relief. I sobbed that day because I realised that being around people who 'got it' had really helped. It was somewhere I could just be, with no agenda. It was a chance to celebrate all the children's achievements. To see them thrive every week and to realise that, actually, life was going to be OK. To see that these people were 'normal' people, was a breath of fresh air. And it might sound like we all sat around discussing DS. We didn't. We ate cake and arranged to have meals out and drink wine. There were two women in particular, Karen and Julia, who both had children the same age as Oscar and both happened to have DS. They became two of my closest and best friends over the years. If you'd had said this would happen to me when I was in that first week after I'd had Oscar, I'd have probably gotten really cross with you, telling you that I didn't need any more friends, especially ones that had kids with DS. The thing is, nine times out of ten, when we meet up, I don't think the words 'Down syndrome' are even mentioned. We're just like every other woman out there with kids, trying desperately to figure out this parenting malarky as we go along. And I love that about our friendship.

The charity also helped to source intervention privately from the beginning for Oscar. Other help was accessed through the NHS (although some of their services were few and far between). People often talk about the fact that our kids are so lucky to have been born in this day and age and not fifty or so years ago when things would have been very different. I'd wanted to try to understand just how different things were now so, when Oscar was around six months old, I started researching. I discovered that if I had left hospital with Oscar in the 1960s, for example, I would have left holding a piece of paper officially deeming him 'uneducable'. I don't even think that's even a word these days! But back then, he would have had no right to an education at all.

I learnt about a lady who had a baby born with DS in the 1950s. She talked of the fact that no one said her child was a 'mongol' (her word) at first, and when they did, it was only when they came to take the baby away to an institution. She'd refused to let her go and her family turned against her as they were deeply ashamed. She brought her home against their wishes and everyone told her she was making a huge mistake. She had a friend who had a baby at the same time, but the friend would never let the children play together because she was frightened that her daughter might catch 'it'. She couldn't go to any coffee mornings or toddler groups for that very same reason. Her child never went to school. She stayed at home all day, every day until she was twelve – when she died.

It seems absolutely unbelievable that it wasn't until the 1971 Education Act that it was decided that no one was 'uneducable' after all and children with Down syndrome started to be entitled to access to learning. At that time people with learning difficulties were categorised as 'educationally subnormal – medium' or 'educationally subnormal – severe' and sent off to an appropriate special school. In 1981 parents were, for the first time, given the opportunity to send their child to a local mainstream school, but that would be unusual and there was little specialist teaching. Schools were given little help. It wasn't until 1995 that the Disability Discrimination Act entitled children with Down syndrome to attend their local mainstream school and not until 2001 that the Special Educational Needs and Disability Act put in place a framework that would actually give the system a chance of working.

Even though the lady who'd had her child in the 1950s brought that little girl home and cared for her, it's devastating to think that she was seen in the eyes of society as worthless. They didn't have the intervention, like we have these days – what possible chance did she have?

I think about the children I was teaching myself; they were all between seven to nine years old and each was a unique person with their own strengths and talents. They rode bikes, they swam, they played rugby, took dance classes ... hey, some of them even skied. That man with DS I had imagined, the one holding hands with his elderly mother and wearing trousers that were far too short for him, is an outdated stereotype and isn't a true indicator of how our children will be living today and in the future. Oscar and his friends have thankfully been born into a world where they are mostly valued and given the opportunities to thrive. I cannot tell you how grateful I am for that.

Over the next couple of months we continued to attend various health checks. There were hearing tests, eye tests, thyroid checks, blood tests and heart check-ups. During that first year it became our new normal, I guess, to visit various hospitals around our local area. We even had a couple of overnight stays due to a severe chest infection and bronchiolitis. But the shock of what unfolded next would knock us for six. Nothing could have prepared us for what was about to happen.

Blog comments

Hi there, I am the mammy of five-month-old Frankie who became very ill after birth and suffered lack of oxygen to the brain. As a result we are facing a possible diagnosis of cerebral palsy in the future. Those early weeks/months were and still are the bleakest of my entire life. While I am getting stronger and realising that Frankie is my son first and foremost and not the condition (I am a midwife by the way and have said those words to parents in the past, not realising I would be telling myself the same advice or realising how hard it is to take that advice), I still find it hard to have hope for the future. I hope in time I am a million miles away from these feelings for Frankie's sake because what hope does he have if I don't have hope for his future, you know? And that adds to my guilt! Anyway, thank you again for sharing your truth with us all.

Heather

Hi, my daughter has shown me your Facebook page and I just wanted to say I can relate to so many things you have written. My son Nick is now thirty-one years old and there has been many ups and downs, as with any child. I just wanted

to share with you where he is now. He lives in
a flat on his own not far from us, he does have
helpers a few hours a day. He works two days
a week, gardening, but his love is cycling. He
rides a tandem and over the last five years has
ridden for charity across Sri Lanka, Madagascar,
Costa Rica and Israel. He has also completed
five London to Brighton cycle rides. This is not
to say how amazing he is, as he certainly has his
moments, but to just say what can be achieved
when people believe and accept him. Like you we
are very proud to have Nick in our family and
only surround ourselves with people who love and
accept him, we come as a package!

Shirley

So I thought you might like to hear how well
my little brother is doing. Sean also has DS, he's
twenty-four. After leaving school he attended a
residential special needs college, he was there for
two years and he did brilliantly. After leaving
he went on to mainstream college and got
qualifications in maths and English. After this
he then started something called Project Choice:
they helped him to get a work placement in an
NHS hospital which lasted for two years and
Sean absolutely loved it. In this time Sean also

moved into supported living, so although there was always someone in the building twenty-four hours a day, he lived in his own flat by himself and it gave him so much independence. He lived on his own for about three years and then decided to move home because he was a little lonely but he did so well. After he finished his work placement in the hospital, his manager had been so impressed with him they interviewed him for a proper paid job and he now works sixteen hours per week in the medical records department and he has been nominated for a national award for all of his hard work and learning. He is amazing – having DS doesn't hold him back, if anything it makes him even more determined, he even recently lost four stone by eating well and going to the gym several times a week. He's a star.

Natasha Hardy

PS: Oscar is absolutely beautiful!

Hello. I've been a fan of your page for a while and love keeping up to date with Oscar's progress and your family's adventures. I saw that today was his first day of big school and wanted to send my best wishes! My beautiful little sister Emily has mosaic Down's [a rarer variant of the condition], is thirteen years old and is fantastic.

(I'm twenty-eight, big age difference!) My mum
and dad have had to fight long and hard to get
her the educational help and support that she
needs but she is doing brilliantly. She went to
mainstream school right up to Y5, when we
decided as a family that special school was better
for her from then on. She has come on in leaps
and bounds recently and, after many years of
being vocal/verbal but not entirely having a two-
way conversation beyond me asking questions
and her answering yes/no, today I called her to
ask how her first day back had gone. She replied
in full story mode to tell me about how she'd
done literacy, play time, numeracy, lunch time,
bingo (which she reliably informs me is a different
type of numeracy!) and told me all about her
new teacher. I still have a huge smile on my face,
hearing how she could talk to me with ease about
her wonderful first day. I guess this seems like a
long way away for you, with Oscar just starting
reception, but I just wanted to let you know that
all the hard work you're putting in with him
now, and all the fights you're taking on to ensure
he gets the best support possible, and all of the
adventures you're forced to let him discover on his
own, will be worth it!

Anon

CHAPTER SIX

'You're the last thing my heart expected.'

Nothing can describe the panic and sheer terror you experience when your baby is going in for heart surgery. Your baby, the baby you're supposed to protect from all the bad stuff in the world, is about to be opened up and operated on.

We were told a machine would take over the job of his heart and lungs for some of the operation. The surgery itself, from start to finish, was predicted to take around four to six hours. A machine though? An *actual machine*? I couldn't get my head around this. What if they lost power and it failed, who'd do the job of the heart and lungs then? (I should note here, I knew they had generators in hospitals and that the likelihood of this happening was very slim, but at this point my mindset was not exactly rational. I was freaking out.) I

77

knew I had to trust the medical professionals as they did this operation every day. But my baby didn't lie on an operating table waiting to be cut open every day and I was scared. So very scared.

Oscar was born with both AVSD and VSD heart defects or, in simpler terms, holes in his heart. Around 40–60 per cent of babies with Down syndrome are born with some form of congenital heart disease. Along with the Down syndrome itself that had been missed at the twenty-week anomaly scan, these conditions also hadn't been detected. Oscar was monitored by his consultant fairly frequently in the months after he was born and in March 2013 we had what we were told was just a precautionary joint appointment with our local hospital and the Royal Brompton Hospital. I remember feeling pretty relaxed that day as Chris, Oscar and I arrived at the hospital. I shouldn't have let my guard down. I've come to learn this over the years because the minute I do, something always seems to knock me for six.

I should have known there was a problem when a large group of consultants and surgeons gathered to stand, staring intently at the screen, while doing an echocardiogram (ECHO) on Oscar. Something about them taking so long and not talking made me feel uneasy. Hushed tones, mumbling under their breath, and then we were ushered into an adjacent room just a few moments afterwards. I knew something wasn't right.

My fears were confirmed: Oscar needed heart surgery imminently. Dr Magee, one of the top cardiologists at the Brompton, explained it all, but honestly? I didn't hear a word. I'd only heard the first sentence. 'Oscar needs open heart surgery.' Tears came. Chris gripped my hand and Oscar sat there completely unfazed by what was unfolding. As the silent tears rolled down my cheek, Dr Magee didn't flinch. Stoic and composed, he ran through facts as he saw them, seemingly oblivious to the outpouring of my emotion.

How could he be so disconnected? I remember thinking. How could he be so nonchalant about it? I knew the answer. He did this sort of thing every day. He had to be neutral.

So, yep, the big one ... open heart surgery. I was told by families who'd also gone through it that the day of the surgery would undoubtedly be the most horrific of my life. They were right. I was told to be prepared for lots of tubes and Oscar being heavily sedated. I was told not to expect to get any sleep myself in the hospital. But I was also told that once it'd been done and it had worked, the prognosis was that he'd have a perfectly normal, functioning heart. Please, please, *please* let it work, I thought.

Now I'm not deeply religious but around this time I found myself silently praying. It kind of went along the lines of, 'Dear God, I know I only ever talk to you when

I need something and I'm really sorry about that, but please let it all be OK.' Shameful of me to admit to only asking for stuff when I really need it but in the interests of this being a personal memoir and thinking it only right to tell the whole truth and nothing but the truth, I thought it best that I be honest.

We were scheduled to go in on the Monday, with the operation itself to take place the next day. Other parents of children who'd been through similar ops had said to me that I wouldn't much feel like it but to get myself out of the hospital and not to sit outside the operating theatre. To go to lunch, to go shopping, but, whatever I did, I wasn't to sit and wait. I needed to keep busy for my own sanity.

I can remember the day my dad drove Chris, Oscar and I up to the Royal Brompton like it was yesterday. It was the second time I'd experienced real panic. The first time was around the time Oscar was born and now, sitting in the back of the car, looking at my boy in his car seat, I felt many of the same feelings. Overwhelming anxiety and loss of control. My chest felt tight, I was talking, trying to remain bright and upbeat, but I felt sick to my stomach. I don't think that feeling of panic left me for a good few days after the operation.

When we arrived at the hospital, we were sent to a ward where they did all their pre-op observations – checking Oscar's oxygen saturation levels, temperature, blood pressure, etc. Oscar had to have an ECHO, an ECG and a chest X-ray, three procedures you'd have thought we were more than used to by now with all the heart appointments he'd had to date but I remained in a state of stress. Chris had stayed with us but, as only one of us was allowed to stay overnight on the ward at Oscar's bedside, he had to go to other accommodation the Brompton had provided.

Around 9.30 p.m. that evening, as I sat alone, watching Oscar sleeping, one of the surgeons visited. He was to be operating on Oscar the following day. He popped his head around the curtain and spoke quietly so as not to wake the babies and children on the ward.

'Hello Mrs Roberts, sorry it's so late. I've just come out of theatre,' he said.

(Um, it's nine-flippin'-thirty! How can you *just* have come out of theatre? You must be knackered. Are you sure you were concentrating on whoever you were operating on? was the monologue going on inside my head.)

'I've come to take you through the operation and all the risks involved.'

(Oh, bloody hell, where's Chris when I need him? I can't do this on my own. Keep calm, Sarah. Hold it together, woman.) 'Yes, of course,' I said.

That's when the magnitude of all this hit me. Sure, consultants had talked the procedure through before and I'd listened intently when other parents had told me what was to happen, but it wasn't really until that moment that I fully understood.

'So, to put it in layman's terms,' he said, 'we sew a patch of man-made surgical material over the hole, stopping the leaky valve.'

(OK, right, that sounds simple enough.)

'Only where we have to sew is very close to a major artery that we can't actually physically see. We know roughly where it is, though.'

(Oh. My. God … he knows '*roughly*'!)

And the conversation went on. I kept quiet. Listening and trying to digest it. But my head was whirling. How could this be happening to us?

The anaesthetist had explained to us earlier that she'd need to administer the general anaesthetic carefully, as babies with DS have atlantoaxial instability (meaning the neck/spine may be poorly developed) and a small trachea (windpipe), meaning that it can be harder to get them to sleep and therefore they could run into problems. Now the surgeon explained the risks in the operation itself – bleeding, infection, irregular heartbeat and damage to the heart, kidneys, liver and/or lungs. Also, if he accidentally sewed the patch in the wrong place and there was damage to the arteries, Oscar might need to have a pacemaker fitted. And, of course, the worst outcome of all was death. It hardly needed to be mentioned, but there it was. The surgeon had said it. 'Death.' *Shit*.

'Mrs Roberts, I'm sure you can appreciate we have to tell you the risks. There's about a three per cent chance that Oscar could die.' Now obviously 3 per cent may not sound that high, right? But that would mean that three babies in every hundred die from the procedure. And something I have touched on already but will get to in more detail later was that our risk of having a baby with Down syndrome had been 1 in 350. Also not high, but we turned out to be that one. So the surgeon would have to forgive me if I wasn't all that confident at this point with the whole statistics thing. He could obviously see it in my face, but it was his next sentence that has stayed with me since and remained very much at the forefront of my mind that night.

'The hole in Oscar's heart has become bigger, Mrs Roberts. We can see from his ECG and ECHO today that it has significantly enlarged since we last saw you. If we don't operate, he might live to see his second birthday – best case scenario his fifth.'

(Don't cry. Don't cry. Do. Not. Cry.)

It was a no-brainer. I took a big, deep breath, gave him a nod to let him know I understood and signed the consent form.

After all that, Oscar's operation turned out to be postponed the following day. He was second on the list but they had run into complications with the sixteen-year-old boy who went down to theatre before him, so they wouldn't get to ours. We were devastated. We had starved our little boy of milk and food since midnight the night before. We had paced the floor with him as he got more and more unhappy, not understanding why he couldn't eat. He was lethargic and weak. And at 3 p.m., when they came to tell us they'd cancelled him for the day, I lost it. I was just so upset. All that build-up. All that worry. And now we were going to have to wait until tomorrow morning. That literally felt like a lifetime away. The surgeon came to see us personally to explain.

Of course, it made perfect sense. The sixteen-year-old's surgery wasn't going well and was taking longer than expected. How wrapped up in us could I be? That could have been Oscar's own surgery that had run into complications. It wasn't and I was so thankful. We gave Oscar some food and milk and within minutes he'd bounced back. That other young man was down on the operating table and I was crying because I'd had a bad day pacing the wards with a hungry baby. It was all that I needed to put things into perspective.

We waited another night.

When morning came I actually felt, for a brief while, an unnerving sense of calm. I think I was just relieved that they had promised me that Oscar would be first down to theatre and that soon all this would be over with. Chris, on the other hand, was not in a great place. He'd been on his own all night. I guess he'd had a lot of time to think. I always knew Chris loved Oscar but it wasn't until that day that I realised to what extent. I don't think I realised just how much I loved our boy either, until then. Previously everything had been about his diagnosis. The big, black cloud of Down syndrome looming over our heads. Now it was about another aspect of our baby boy's health. His life. It wasn't until I experienced the prospect of losing him – and understood that it didn't bear thinking about – that I truly got that.

They knew that Oscar was going down first, so they'd given him a drug that prepared him for sedation. By the time that Chris came onto the ward that morning, Oscar was very sleepy. Chris sat by his bed and watched him. Neither of us were talking, nothing more needed to be said. I watched as tears silently rolled down Chris's cheeks. And there it was. Love. All-encompassing love. A father's love for his first-born son, mixed with uncontrollable, unimaginable fear.

Eventually, the anaesthetist came to take us down. We were allowed to be with Oscar until he went under and one of us was to hold him until then. I've talked about it before, but when we were in the NICU with Oscar after he was born, I had this overwhelming sense of wanting to pick him up and run. Out of the door, to the end of the corridor, out the hospital and just keep running. It was before we'd had the blood test back confirming he had Down syndrome, so in my head at that moment, if I ran, I would never have known or had to deal with the diagnosis. Here I was now, my baby about to be operated on, and I wanted to run again. Of course, I knew I couldn't but that feeling set in again. Loss of control. I will never forget the moment they put him under. The panic in his eyes, the struggle, Oscar looking up at Chris who was losing it at the other end of the room, me looking back down at my baby, his eyes wide, staring back at me. *What are they doing to me, Mummy? Help me, Mummy*. And then a gasp. The dire-smelling gas had filled his lungs. He was asleep. They'd told us they'd call my mobile when he was back up in paediatric intensive care. That might not be for up to six hours ... then the door closed behind us.

The hours passed in a blur. I know we got out of the hospital. I know we ate breakfast somewhere and wandered aimlessly around the shops. But can I remember any conversation the two of us had? I think we both went through moments of needing to talk about the most irrelevant crap, to moments of silence. My phone kept beeping with messages from family and friends that morning. They were obviously all checking we were OK and wanting updates of what was going on. And with every beep, I jumped. I will never forget where I was when the hospital called four-and-a-half hours after we left Oscar. Right next to the cold sesame noodles with vegetables at the deli counter in Whole Foods (we were attempting to get lunch and anyone who knows my husband will know that Whole Foods presents far too much choice for him to make a quick decision).

It had only been four and a half hours – I thought it was supposed to take up to six? Something's happened. Something's happened to him. I froze. 'I can't answer it, you answer it, Chris.' He did. After all that open-heart surgery, Oscar was OK. The operation had been a success. He was being transferred to the paediatric intensive care unit (PICU) shortly and we were to go back to the hospital waiting room to be called to see him. We felt so relieved. He was still in intensive care, we weren't out of the woods yet, but … it had been a success. I needed to see him. I needed to be back at the hospital. I didn't want to wait while Chris paid for his teriyaki beef stir-fry. I needed to see my baby now.

Obviously we made it back well before they called us in. I remember sitting in the waiting room, Chris eating his beef, and seeing a team of about eight nurses, doctors and hospital porters, pushing monitors, machines and a bed, past the window. In that bed was Oscar. He must have flashed past in about two seconds but I knew it was him. He was just lying there, lifeless. I mean obviously he wasn't lifeless, he was asleep and still under general anaesthetic but it hurt – it *really* hurt – to see him like that.

Eventually we were called in. People were right when

they said that nothing could ever have prepared me for the moment I saw my baby lying there, attached to goodness knows how many machines and monitors. Eyes closed and so still. My heart felt like it was breaking at that moment. Oscar had an endotracheal tube in his mouth that went down into his windpipe to provide an airway. He was on a respirator to help with his breathing. He had central IV lines leading to a vein that in turn fed to his right atrium. Their purpose was to monitor central heart pressures and give fluids and medications. An arterial line, which is a small tube in an artery, measured his blood pressure and oxygen levels. He had two chest tubes going into the space between the chest wall and the lung, an area known as pleural space. These had been placed after the heart surgery to prevent the accumulation of bodily fluids. The chest tubes drained air, blood and fluid from his chest cavity. He had a catheter and was being administered oxygen through a mask. His heart was being monitored for its rhythm, BPM rate and respiratory rate. He looked a mess. Chris and I, even though we thought we had prepared ourselves for the moment we saw him, were not expecting him to look the way he did. I didn't cry when I saw him. I think I must have been in shock.

Oscar had one-to-one ratio care in PICU and we could not have been more grateful to the amazing team of doctors and nurses who looked after him when he was in there. They were, to say the very least, incredible. They were not only attentive and caring towards Oscar but to us as well. They made sure we understood what was going on, alleviated our fears and concerns and tried so very hard to distract us with chat as we watched on. Anyone who has had the misfortune of sitting in an ICU will know how scary it is. Machines beep loudly, alarms go off, parents sit silently by the bedside, just staring … for hours … Oscar was in the bed next to the sixteen-year-old who'd had surgery the day before (he was doing well, thankfully) but our baby looked so tiny in comparison. I would have done anything to swap places with him right there and then.

I find it hard to recall in the right order the events of the next few days. I know that when Oscar woke up he was very upset. We were told he wouldn't be able to feel pain but they couldn't control his panic with a drug. I knew Oscar and I could see he was scared. That first evening, they took out the tube opening up his airway. Chris was with him when they did this as it was about midnight and, after the emotion of the day, I was told to go and get some sleep. This was when they saw that he was breathing on his own. I'd waited for Chris to come back to the room, unable to relax until I knew Oscar was OK. Once I knew all was well, for the first time in days, I allowed myself to properly fall asleep.

We were there the next morning and stayed late into

the evening. We only left Oscar to grab some food or get some fresh air. We sat there for days, just watching. It's incredible how quickly children fight their way back. I remember being allowed to give him some milk from the bottle on the second day and how proud I was of him for coping so well. Just little things like this were a step forward in getting out of there. On day three, his chest drains were taken out. We thought all was well but it turned out, when they did a chest X-ray, that he had a collapsed lung (pneumothorax). When they'd taken the drains out, air had gotten into the space around the lung. This build-up of air was putting pressure on the lung, so it couldn't expand as much as it normally does when you take a breath. A setback. It meant that Oscar would have to stay in PICU longer as he needed to be given oxygen to help the lung. We were so gutted. We had literally been told that morning that we'd be moving to the ward later that day, but now we were to stay in intensive care. Obviously, it was for the best but it was still really hard. They did say, however, that they couldn't quite believe at this point how well Oscar was doing, sitting up and smiling, when there was so much strain on his lung.

So we stayed in PICU a few more days and were eventually moved to the ward for a couple more nights. I was anxious the first night on the ward. He was no longer on a one-to-one ratio of care, with a nurse watching him. Just little old me. What if something happened in the night? I was the one who had to look after him now. That first night on the ward I didn't sleep, I just watched over Oscar as he slept.

After ten long days we were discharged. The relief was immense. We'd already seen a bit of a change in Oscar's energy levels but as the months passed we were astounded by the difference in him. We likened it to him being a Duracell bunny. Before this, I don't think we realised just how much of a struggle everything was for him. He just used to sit and play with toys, sometimes not turning to us if we called him. As soon as he'd recovered from the op, it seemed like he had a new set of those Duracell batteries. His colour changed, he looked healthier and happier, and he was off bum-shuffling everywhere. When once his breathing had always been quicker and laboured, now he seemed calm.

We couldn't thank the Royal Brompton Hospital enough for the surgery and the continued care Oscar had – and is continuing to receive. He was obviously still closely monitored but after check-ups at two, four and six months after the surgery, he went to yearly checks. Oscar was and is a bright, confident and strong little boy, and I truly believe that without that surgery, he wouldn't be. Many children with Down syndrome in the past were institutionalised and they were often deprived of all but the most elementary medical services.

Fortunately, there have been major improvements in the healthcare provision during the past twenty years and we are so thankful that Oscar was born in the 2010s, when people with DS are given the same care as you and I. His precious life is worth everything to us and we will be forever grateful.

Blog comments

Hi there. Our eight-month-old son, Theo, was born in November last year and after a very traumatic birth, we were advised that Theo has Down syndrome. He was very poorly when born and spent three weeks on the neonatal unit having chemotherapy at just four days old for TAM [transient abnormal myelopoiesis, a bone-marrow disorder that can occur in newborns who have Down syndrome]. Theo has made a remarkable recovery and is now developing marvellously, both physically and socially/emotionally. Theo will need a heart operation when he gets to eighteen months, but until then, we are excited to see how he continues to develop. He is such an amazing little boy and we feel so blessed. We often read about Oscar's journey and love seeing his development. As he is a bit older than Theo, it's great to see the various stages that we have coming up. Thank you for sharing with us. All the very best.

Emma Thomas Payn

Hi, Sarah, we have been waiting for my son, Alex, to get a date for a complete AVSD repair. We hadn't even had the pre-op so I felt like there was a safe enough distance for me to read your experiences. Well, of course, we were brought in for his pre-op on Tuesday then called on Wednesday to bring him in for surgery on Friday. So here we are on the night before and I am terrified and as you say, heartbroken. My gorgeous boy, I don't want them to touch him but I know it has to be done.

Emily Turner

My older sister has Down syndrome and had two major open-heart ops aged seven and eleven (at the time they couldn't operate on babies). My sister is still going strong at thirty-seven having yearly check-ups. The docs never know what to expect as she basically is the statistic for that sort of operation. At the time my dad (not a violent man in the slightest!) actually held a doctor against the wall after he suggested they wouldn't operate on my sister and that the kindest thing would be to let her die! So the first op of its kind, really, at Great Ormond Street and she is still doing brilliantly. I'm a passionate believer that people with Down's have so much to give which is why I love reading your blog.

Beth Dunnett

Noah had open heart surgery at ten months old. It was literally the hardest day of our lives yet it is such a humbling experience that we will never forget. We were amazed by the surgeon who would come in and see all the beautiful little babies at the weekend in his tracksuit. He was a true inspiration, had so much love for his job and I just knew we could put our trust in him. I'll never forget that man. He was so humble. I remember just saying, 'Thank you' a million times and he just said, 'Please, no need to thank me'. But you never quite feel like you could ever repay them. We have Noah's heart check-up coming up soon, all been good so far. What would we do without these amazing people?! To think forty or fifty years ago our children probably wouldn't have made it.

Sharon Jones

CHAPTER SEVEN

'Ignore the noise and follow your own choice.'

I didn't tell you in the previous chapter that while Oscar's heart surgery had been going on, I was actually around twelve weeks pregnant. Contrary to how it might sound, falling pregnant with my second, when my first was just seven and a half months old, was the plan.

The baby I'm talking about is Oscar's younger brother, Alfie. The age gap between them is just sixteen and a half months, which is probably a tad smaller than we'd anticipated (I'm sure I said something to Chris along the lines of, 'We better start trying as these things can take forever'). But we did really want another baby and were so grateful that we'd been fortunate enough to fall pregnant straight away.

When Chris and I had first gotten serious and had started talking marriage, babies and so on, we both had said we'd quite like three children. We're both from families of three, you see. I have two sisters and Chris has a brother and sister so maybe that's why we were keen on the idea. But when we had Oscar, we felt strongly that we really wanted him to have siblings and for them to be close in age if they could be.

I guess there are usually two trains of thought. There are the people, like us, that want their child to have that close support network. To have a sibling (or siblings) so that they'll show them how it's done. To always have a friend, I suppose. Then there are the other types, who I totally respect by the way, who say that after having their child with DS, they don't want any more, as they'd rather focus all their time and energy on that child. I'm not sure there is a right or wrong answer. Being in the thick of things now with three small children aged five and under, I'd say there's a lot to be said for having just one. I spend an awful lot of time worrying that I'm not devoting enough time to any of them, let alone Oscar, but then watching them together, their bond and seeing how much Oscar has developed, I think having siblings has played a big part in the little person he has become today. 'Mum guilt' is tough at times though.

When I fell pregnant the first time, the future was full of all sorts of hopes and dreams. Such a special time. The second time was different and full of mixed emotions. So very happy that we were fortunate enough to fall pregnant again. Excited, particularly for Oscar, that he'd have a baby brother or sister to grow up with. But, equally, that period was tinged with apprehension and uncertainty. Would all be well with this baby? Would the birth be as traumatic as last time? Could I do it all over again, without the naivety and innocence I'd had before?

It's my belief that there are always going to be those women out there, whether they've had a baby with DS or not, who are simply happy to be having a baby and don't feel any need to screen or to have any sort of testing, whether that be a blood test or invasive testing (such as an amnio or CVS – chorionic villus sampling) in their pregnancies. They feel this way because the outcome would be completely irrelevant. These same women also say that having a baby with DS or any other chromosome abnormality wouldn't create a viable reason to terminate. They morally and ethically disagree with screening and testing.

Then there are those women who, without any question or doubt, categorically state they wouldn't want a baby with DS so would want to know to have the option to have an abortion. These are the women who feel the need to have screening and if their result was higher than anticipated (1 in 150 chance or lower), they potentially might go on to have a definitive test and if they flag up as a positive, they will then abort. There are also the women who choose a NIPT (Non-

Invasive Prenatal Test – such as the Harmony test) who again wait on those results and based on them, may or may not go ahead with an abortion (I should point out here the Harmony or other NIPTs are not definitive. It's still only 99 per cent accurate). Not forgetting the women who are screened and, finding the result comes back as high risk (for example a 1 in 23 chance that the baby will have DS), will then proceed with an abortion without finding out for sure whether the baby has the condition. A woman does this assuming that her child may or may not have Down syndrome, but she doesn't want to take that chance.

It's such a hugely sensitive and emotive subject and one that I try very hard not to pass judgement on. We all feel very differently and I wouldn't even begin to tell someone how they should think or feel. I respect that the way everyone approaches this differently is their very personal choice. But you see, the thing is, I strongly believe that if there was more balanced information out there about DS, about what it means to have a baby with DS today, I don't think the abortion rate would be quite so high. As it stands at the moment, around 90 per cent of women who find out they're expecting a baby with DS, choose to terminate. Now, don't get me wrong, hearing about Down syndrome can be a huge shock, it's not the outcome any of us expect but it breaks my heart to think of terminating a baby on the basis they have DS.

I hope that when I share my personal account, people will respect the decisions I made. They were, after all, decisions I made for my own emotional well-being. Call it what you like … I call it self-preservation. I remember telling my best friend fairly soon after we'd had Oscar that we'd like another baby and her asking, quite candidly, was I having another baby to make up for any kind of failings I had felt with Oscar? I should be clear that she was asking how I felt, not because she was suggesting or has ever thought Oscar was anything less than perfect. And I remember quite vividly at the time saying no, I didn't feel that way. But on reflection, looking back now, I think perhaps I did feel like I'd failed. I definitely thought I'd failed Chris, my family and his family. I'd wished after Oscar had been born that I could have just given them the son, grandson, nephew and cousin they'd all been longing for. I imagined nobody else wanted DS at that point any more than I did. The ironic thing? Chris has never felt anything other than love towards Oscar. He's really OK with the DS. Always has been and always will be. And our family? They couldn't love this kid more. It was me, again. My issues with DS and my issues with striving for the perfect child or what I imagined the perfect child to be back then.

If I'm honest, in those first few weeks with Oscar, in the depths of feeling like I was grieving the loss of a child (ridiculous to even think now), I thought that another child might make me feel better. But as my second pregnancy went on I understood that when Oscar was born, I had worried I wouldn't love him. I didn't feel that sudden rush of love that so many people talk about. It took me a little while to truly love Oscar. As it turned out, the ironic thing was that by the time Alfie was born, I actually worried I wouldn't love him *as much* as I loved Oscar. Life has a habit of coming full circle.

When it came to Alfie, there was no greater chance that I might have another baby with DS than there was for the next person. There are three types of Down syndrome: trisomy 21 (nondisjunction), translocation and mosaicism. Oscar had the most common, trisomy 21, which doesn't pass from parent to child through the genes. When I fell pregnant with Alfie, I was offered an appointment to see a screening midwife. I had decided to go back to the same hospital where I'd had Oscar, although I really didn't fully know how I felt about this. They had been amazing with Oscar when he'd been in NICU. They'd looked after us both so well. They knew me and my background and I was familiar with them. But on the flip side, I knew that going back there would bring back some pretty raw memories. Perhaps I'd have felt better going somewhere completely new? And as much as I knew that the screening I'd had with Oscar wasn't definitive, I still felt like my faith in them had been dented a little. They hadn't picked up on the DS or the two holes in Oscar's heart. Could they miss something again?

At my twelve-week scan with Oscar, we opted to take combined screening. I say 'opted' because I very clearly remember being handed the form and signing it, but I don't ever remember any of it being explained. I got the impression that this was just protocol. That everyone opted to have the screening and that me having it was what was supposed to happen. And although I recall a midwife taking my bloods, there was no chat about the results and what might happen if they weren't what we'd hoped for. Equally, there was no attempt to find out if we even understood the impact of screening itself. I was thirty-three years old at the time. The combined screening test measures the nuchal translucency (from scanning the baby) and two pregnancy hormones called PAPP-A and hCG (Pregnancy-Associated Plasma Protein-A and human Chorionic Gonadotropin, taken from the mother through a blood test). This information is combined with the mother's age and the gestation of the baby to get a result. We were sent a letter a few days after our scan, letting us know that we were low 'risk' (not considered likely to have a baby with DS) and that our odds were 1 in 350. You are considered high risk if you have 1 in 150 or lower chance. I remember receiving the letter and thinking that it was obviously fine if we were in this category and genuinely didn't give it too much thought after that.

With Alfie – and I'm presuming because I had Oscar on my record – I was offered a CVS (chorionic villus sampling). This procedure is usually carried out between weeks eleven and fourteen of pregnancy and involves a needle being inserted through the abdomen. A sample of cells are removed from the placenta (the organ linking the mother's blood supply with her unborn baby) and tested. I was told that I could have my twelve-week scan, get my odds (whether I had a low or high chance of having a baby with DS) and go from there. If we then felt we wanted the CVS, they would rush us up to St George's Hospital in London.

At my scan I'm sure they were being especially nice to me, as they were able to give me my odds there and then. I'd had a blood sample taken the week before. Along with the measurement of the foetus, the nuchal fold, the test showed my odds with Alfie of having DS were 1 in 4,400. Despite me having had Oscar and despite me now being that little bit older, the results this time were significantly better than last.

It was around this time I recalled a friend's wise words of wisdom and his brilliant analogy. With Oscar we had had a 1 in 350 chance of having a baby with DS. With Alfie, this time, we had a 1 in 4,400. It came back to that red dot at the bottom of the cup again. Out of all the cups, first time round, we'd picked the one cup that had had the red dot on it, right? (That was Oscar.) This time I now had 4,400 cups in front of me and again only one cup with a red dot on it. So, what really were the chances of me picking *that* cup? You'd have to be pretty unlucky, hey? Or lucky, it depends how you look at it. I mean, if I'd have gotten a dot in the bottom of my cup again, I'd more than certainly have to start doing the lottery!

At both my twelve- and twenty-week scans with Alfie, I noticed that they took a great deal more time looking at and measuring the baby on their screen. Were they being careful to cover all bases? Had I been unlucky last time with my sonographers? Were they just being thorough? Or perhaps they'd read my notes and realised that, less than a year previously, I'd been scanned and they hadn't picked up any issues. What do you reckon?

As it turned out, a few days after my scan we were going in again, for the heart surgery that I described in the previous chapter, so a CVS was literally the last thing on my mind. There was no way I could fit it in, both timing wise or emotionally so it wasn't up for debate. I would sit on it for a while and ponder my options.

It was now the summer of 2013 and there was also a new blood test available, only offered in two top London clinics. It had been discovered that a blood sample taken from the mother at any time from early pregnancy can be analysed for cell-free fetal DNA, which is essentially a marker in the mother's blood of the DNA of the baby. The result of the simple blood test, taken at ten weeks or later, can predict to more than 99 per cent accuracy Down syndrome, 98 per cent Edwards syndrome and 80 per cent Patau syndrome. I did my research and I listened to professionals marvel over this new test – but something didn't sit right with me. It was still only 99 per cent conclusive. This wasn't a definitive test. There was still a chance that you'd pay all that money to have it done and it mightn't be accurate. And with us being that 'one' that had had the baby with DS, I couldn't put my faith in it personally.

The other option available to me was an amniocentesis. An amnio is usually carried out during weeks fifteen to twenty of pregnancy, when a needle is used to extract a sample of the amniotic fluid that surrounds the foetus in the womb. It would be examined and tested for a number of conditions. Whether or not to have the test was probably one of the hardest decisions I've ever had to make in my life. And by sharing my account of what happened, I don't mean to influence or to dissuade. It's obviously a very controversial and delicate subject that, as I said, I believe is every individual's personal choice but, in the end, I decided to have an amnio.

It's something I don't think I regret doing but something I'm aware I'm not altogether comfortable with admitting out loud. I have friends who've gone on to have another child, after having a child with DS, who haven't felt the need to know if their unborn baby had DS. So why did I? If I loved Oscar with every inch of my body like I said I did by this point, would it be so terrible to have another child with DS? It wouldn't, for the record, and I'm pretty certain I wouldn't have done anything about it had I been told that Alfie had DS, too, but for me, right then, it was a case of being prepared and I couldn't risk losing control of a situation again, as I had done when they told me about Oscar.

I have heard about some of the other disorders a child can be born with and, with those in mind, I believe that DS was probably the least of my worries. An amnio can't test for everything so, with hindsight, was I risking the life of my unborn child only for him to be born with a different complication? Maybe the fact that I was having the test would mean that karma would come back and bite me and he'd be starved of oxygen and have brain damage during birth.

All these thoughts played through my mind in the lead-up to the procedure. I thought about other things, too. I'd had friends of mine who'd struggled to get pregnant. Some that still haven't been able to many years on and some that devastatingly never will. I've known of others that have had IVF, who I know wouldn't even contemplate for one single second risking anything happening to their unborn child but, deep in the pit of my stomach, I knew that I had to go through with this. That I couldn't go through the next six months not knowing. I felt bad though. I felt guilty. But I needed to know.

Some people are morally opposed to the screening because the test can be a catalyst for people deciding to terminate their pregnancies, should it flag up something as 'wrong', which I really do understand, but this was my decision and I remained strong in how I felt. Up until the morning of the amnio, I still wasn't a hundred per cent sure if I'd actually go through with it. Chris had always said it was ultimately my decision and that he'd support me whatever I decided to do but it wasn't something I was taking lightly. I thought long and hard about my unborn child. I thought about the consequences of my actions. But in the end, I went ahead and had the procedure done. It wasn't painful. Just a little uncomfortable. But to this day, I still feel like I betrayed Oscar.

My mum and Oscar had been waiting for me outside. I was told to go home and take it easy for the next forty-eight hours. I wasn't allowed to drive or to lift Oscar and I can honestly say that for the two days that followed, wondering if I'd put my unborn baby's life at risk, I was riddled with guilt. A few days later, we were called to say all was OK. I cried when I put the phone down. Not because I was relieved, but because, sitting next to me, my little boy was smiling up at me, so blissfully unaware of what I'd done. So completely in love with his mummy. How could I not want another Oscar? I thought, and the tears fell.

When Alfie was born without complication, I felt guilty again. An emotion that hit me like a ton of bricks, for it was an emotion that I hadn't banked on in this situation. I assumed I'd feel this rush of love that everyone had talked about. That when Alfie was born, I'd feel all the things that everyone else claimed they felt when they had had their babies. I knew I'd missed out on so much with Oscar because I was too wrapped up in his diagnosis to really just look at the baby in my arms and love him like he desperately needed me to. I felt guilty that we'd always said we wanted more children but lying there now in my hospital bed (opposite the one I'd been lying in when we'd found out about Oscar, by the way), I was now thinking that it wasn't fair on Oscar, that he'd now have to share his mummy and daddy.

I'd had the elective caesarean that I'd been adamant I wanted because I couldn't in my mind accept that something might not go wrong this time. I needed calm. I needed to be in control. And I had been … it was everything I'd needed it to be. But, actually, when all was said and done, this time I was fighting my own demons. I'd felt guilty that I'd brought Alfie in to the world so soon, when Oscar still depended on me so much. I felt cheated that I didn't immediately feel that rush of love for my second-born, the way others had told me I would.

And mostly I felt guilty for thinking that having Alfie, my supposed 'perfect child', would make me feel more of a mother than I had the first time around. That first time, I felt, I had let down those I loved.

Of course, all these feelings were very short-lived. The guilt left me and seeing the boys together I knew we'd done the right thing. Oh, and the love came, too. Just not in the gushy rush that everyone talked about. When it came, it came in abundance though. But looking back, I think it's important to note that every mother out there rarely feels the same when she has a new baby. Whether she gives birth unexpectedly to a baby with DS. Whether she gives birth to a child without complications. We all feel so very differently and I'm here to say that I really think that's OK to admit.

Blog comments

Sorry to bother you but I want to thank you for being an inspiration. Like you and your family my partner and I have an eight-week-old son named Max who was diagnosed with Down syndrome after birth. I had all my screening tests and was 'low risk'. Like you, I thought my world had ended and have blamed myself for my gorgeous little boy having Down's. We have always wanted to give Max a sibling and I have now been frightened that the chances of another child having Down's would be increased. When my friend showed me your page and I read your blogs and looked at your pictures (your little boy is gorgeous!) it was lovely to see that what I've been feeling is natural and that things are not all dark and gloomy and in fact can and will be OK.

Kirstie Sharp

Hello. I am the mother of a beautiful eight-month-old girl called Olivia Rose. She makes me so proud. I am one of these mums that won't let doctors tell me my child is different and won't do things. Olivia has had my one hundred per cent attention for the whole eight months. I spend hours teaching her things, playing with her, helping her learn and so far everything I have done has paid off. She is advanced in all her motor skills: from seven months she was sitting, rolling and trying to crawl. I could not be any prouder of her if I tried. We shocked her physio, it was an amazing feeling, but recently I have been thinking I would like another child. The reason behind this is I want her to have a close bond with a sibling; the closer the age gap, I think, the better this bond would be. Also, I hope the sibling would look after her and protect her. I wondered if you had a close age gap with your children and if you think this helps the development of children with DS. I will do anything for Olivia to help her progress. Then I get doubts – will it be too much hard work? Will it impact on Olivia in a bad way? She won't have me one hundred per cent. Will people think I tried for another baby so soon because I'm not happy with Olivia? All these things play on my mind. I just needed to talk to someone who may possibly understand. Thank you.

Suzanna Miller

We had Bethany after having Archie who graced us with his extra chromosome. I was terrified, not of DS but of the unknown. We weren't aware Archie would have DS so the diagnosis was a complete shock. I suffer with anxiety anyway, so we decided to pay for the Harmony test (the new NIPT) just to know either way. There was no way we were going to even consider termination. If our third pregnancy meant another child with Down syndrome our lives wouldn't change, we already had Archie and he made us 'experts' in all that is DS. We just wanted to be prepared so that my anxiety didn't get worse through pregnancy but only because of the unknown.

Becky Carless

CHAPTER EIGHT

'Think before you speak. Read before you think.'
– FRAN LEBOWITZ, TIPS FOR TEENS,
SOCIAL STUDIES, 1981

When we brought Alfie home from hospital, Oscar was just over sixteen months old. Oscar was doing OK developmentally but the gap between him and his mainstream peers was definitely starting to show more. Each milestone was taking him just that little bit longer to master. Rolling over, sitting up, crawling (he didn't do this for ages, preferring to bottom-shuffle) and self-feeding all happened eventually, but each time it always felt like we were waiting just a tad longer than everyone else. The thing is, if you're a parent of a child with Down syndrome or have, like me, worked with a child with additional needs, you know that success happens a little bit, every single day. Albeit in very tiny, baby steps, but it does happen. I learnt that this was true of Oscar. That the things that might not be such a big deal with typically developing children become the biggest triumph imaginable for Oscar.

Take, for example, the self-feeding thing. Oscar began to put his spoon in his yoghurt pot, take a spoonful and attempt to put in in his mouth. He wouldn't quite complete it, preferring to wave the spoon around, splodges of said yoghurt hurtling their way across the kitchen. We would just be super-chuffed because the previous week he hadn't even thought about putting the spoon in the pot.

There is no such thing as a typical child with Down syndrome. Our children are as different from each other as are all children. There are, of course, books and information online which list when the average child with DS is likely to sit alone or stand, but I used to try to avoid them. I do remember, when I was waiting for Oscar to start walking and feeling a little sad that he was still a way off, that I googled, 'When does a child with DS usually walk?' The answer was it could potentially be anywhere from thirteen to forty-eight months. I mean, who knew the window would be so large? I felt fairly disheartened. People often say that children grow up too fast, but I guess when it came to Oscar we've never really had that experience.

Alfie was born just before Christmas 2013 and the

following Valentine's Day, at nineteen months, Oscar started walking independently. It was, in its simplicity, success in its purest and most beautiful form. We'd waited a long time (although I do know that, by comparison with other children his age who happen to have DS, we weren't waiting as long as some). But in that moment, I genuinely felt like my heart might burst with pride.

It was around this time that I decided to start writing the blog I called 'Don't Be Sorry'. As I've said previously, when Oscar was about to go in to have his heart surgery, I remember feeling this sudden urge to start writing some things down. I called it my therapy as for some reason it felt like I could make sense of things if I wrote it all down but, as a bonus, as I continued to write and post publicly, it seemed to help others in a similar position to us. Not only that, but people who had no affiliation to Down syndrome were interested in hearing about Oscar. Hearing about a family who potentially looked slightly different from theirs, they wanted to learn more about it all.

I think some of my most-viewed posts over the years have been about some of the ridiculous things people have said or indirectly said to us and as I opened up about our encounters (remember the story about the GP who called Oscar a 'medical student's dream' with all his associated health issues), I realised that other people would share their experiences, too. Sharing stories helped raise awareness, yes, but it also became an outlet for other people to vent. Oh, and over the years there have been some right clangers.

Walking back to Waterloo station after a hen party in London, I got chatting to one of the other girls. We didn't actually know each other, but we were both friends of the hen and when I say she was a girl, I would hazard a guess that she was probably a woman in her late thirties or early forties. We'd been talking a while as we walked and then the conversation switched inevitably, as these things often do when you have children, to my life with Oscar. We talked about how he was doing, how having had Alfie recently, it'd been so lovely to see the bond develop between the boys, and then onto the fact that he'd had heart surgery. Hers was typical of most people's reactions when they hear a ten-month baby boy has just undergone open heart surgery – she gasped and commented on how awful that must have been for both us and him and as usual I replied with, 'Yes, it was probably one of the most horrific experiences of my life.' She nodded in agreement and asked how the heart was now, again not an unusual response. I told her that he was still needing six-monthly check-ups so they could keep an eye on things but by all intents and purposes, he now had a perfectly normal functioning heart.

'Amazing,' she said, 'just incredible.' Then she asked, 'And the Down syndrome?'

Puzzled, I said, 'What do you mean?' (If that looks rude written down, by the way, I didn't say it like that. I genuinely didn't have a clue what she meant.)

'The Down syndrome ... so, is that cured now, too?'

Yep.

She actually said that.

Word for word.

Now, I don't doubt for a minute that she's a wonderful lady. But what a comment, from someone I can only imagine is a well-educated, well-respected woman. She's just asked me if my son's Down Syndrome had now been cured.

REALLY?

You couldn't make this stuff up.

I was in Waitrose a while back (I appreciate that may make me sound posh – I can assure you we don't do our weekly shops in there, it's more that it's the most convenient place to whizz in and out with a toddler and a baby in tow) and a lovely cashier lady took a particular interest in Oscar. She asked me his name, his age, etc. She was lovely. I mean truly lovely. Then she dropped this on me: 'We have quite a few of those that come in here.'

Now by 'those' I'm guessing she was referring to people with DS. But again, really? THOSE?! Perhaps this was the point when I should have put her in her place and told her just how annoying her comment was. But instead, I just smiled and thanked her for my shopping before we went on our way.

I'm often asked where Oscar is 'on the spectrum'. Is this any different to asking anyone how smart their child is? I understand that the questioner is usually well-meaning, so I (gently) try to explain that it's really not the 'done thing' to ask such a question. Just as you probably wouldn't ask a parent about the intelligence of their offspring, this is just not something ever to ask of someone who happens to have DS. Like the rest of us, of course, people with Down syndrome have different levels of intelligence but I much prefer the question, 'So how's he getting on?' as it tells me that they're kind of asking the same sort of thing in not so many words but it doesn't feel so blatant.

One of my favourite stories of all time – though it's not a nice one; in fact, when I tell it, people are usually horrified – comes again from a friend of a friend, who asked me, in a very loud voice at a party, 'Are there any indications of just how mentally retarded he is?'

I felt those around us shuffle nervously, looking at the floor, probably as shocked and dumfounded as I was. At the time, Oscar was under a year old, I was pregnant with Alfie and I didn't have the strength to say anything, other than how great he was doing, but I was honestly completely floored by this person. I wonder what might be my reaction to this question now, all these years later. Would I have the strength to put her in her place? I'm pretty certain I would. I just simply can't fathom how people are *still* saying such ridiculous things.

I guess people are always going to say and do things that are out of your control. As time went on and as I got stronger, whether that be as a mum to Oscar and all that came with the DS or just being a mum to two little ones, I realised that you can get cross or get upset or you can gently educate as you go along. A thick skin is often required; if you challenge every single thing everyone says or does in life, you'd be forever fighting. I think perhaps having DS in our lives has given me a different perspective. I've definitely become fiercely protective, knowing that I'm probably going to have to look out for my little man for the rest of my life.

I'll never forget a conversation I had with Oscar's cousin Bella. Bella is slightly older than Oz (our nickname for Oscar) and this particular conversation took place when she was just four years old. I've always thought that Bella was fairly advanced in her speech and wise beyond her age. It was around this time that my sister Clare had signed Bella up for ballet classes. Shortly after they started, Clare told that me Bella no longer wanted to go. I asked her why she'd given up ballet classes and didn't she want to become a dancer like her auntie Sarah used to be? Her response was, 'No, it made my legs boring and I got out of breath quite a lot.' (To be fair, this was a very valid point. Dancing does hurt your legs and is pretty knackering.) Anyway, I found it heart-warming that, although Oscar couldn't necessarily answer Bella when she asked him a question, she never tired of him and they always seemed to find a way to communicate, usually through hugs and a lot of laughter.

I asked my sister if Bella understood about Oscar not being able to talk that well, which he couldn't at that point, and she replied, 'She often now notices people who have Down syndrome and will say, "He or she is just like Oscar, aren't they, Mummy?" And when I say, yes and what is it that Oscar has, she doesn't say Down syndrome, she always says "Magic" because he's just that extra bit special, isn't he?'

When Clare told me this my eyes welled up with tears. I know some of you will say that he's no different to you or me, or that we shouldn't label him or differentiate, but I really liked Bella's way of putting it. For he *is* magic. And she's right. He really *is* just that little bit extra-special. I just loved that she saw that, accepted him, loved him and didn't for one second see anything wrong with having a little bit of magic in her life. As the old saying goes, perhaps the world really would be a happier place if we could all see the world through the eyes of a child.

I'd like to point out that most of the time, in our experience, people are amazing. Like I've said previously, I'm sure people don't mean to say/do such ridiculous or hurtful things. I guess it's them not knowing what to say (I'd like to point out that at times I can be just as much of a numpty, putting my foot in it when talking to other people). So, am I gonna change? Become one of these confrontational, hard-nosed mothers who put people in their places? Probably not. I think I'll just sit quietly, happy in the knowledge that they don't have any clue what it's actually like to have the magic of my little boy Oscar in their lives. And if you've ever known anyone with a disability or a difference, I suspect you know exactly what I'm talking about.

Blog comments

Honey, I just wanted to say your blogs are keeping me company on my train journeys and I'm just in awe of you all. They are just beautiful and I'm speechless really. You should put them all in a book; anyway, I hope we cross paths someday and I get to meet your inspirational family.

Kerry Ellis (West End Star)

Hi, Sarah. I'm Bess. I was at Sheffield Children's Hospital with my little boy Amos yesterday and

one of the consultants told me about your blog.
On 4 January I gave birth to my second child,
my little boy. In pregnancy they knew that my
child had small limbs but they didn't know why.
As I had been low risk for DS, they had ruled
that out but nothing else made sense. On the 7th,
they diagnosed him with DS. I know that feeling
you had when you received news about Oscar. It
subsided reasonably quickly when we realised this
was an exciting adventure that were honoured to
be on. I know some times will be hard but at this
stage we have no idea how the DS will affect his
development. I want to thank you for your blog,
your honesty and the smile it brings to my face.
I'm excited to see where this journey will take my
little family and I look forward to seeing more
about your beautiful boy Oscar.
Thank you.

Bess Popplewell

Hi, I just want to say thank you for your page as
it has really helped me. I love reading your stories
and you have three beautiful children. Olivia was
born on 15 July 2016 and is eight weeks old. We
were told she might have trisomy 21 on the 16th
and it was confirmed on the 20th. I can honestly
say I felt just how you described it and I didn't

know how I was going to cope. I already have a four-year-old little boy so I had to be strong. I feel so much more positive now and you have been a huge part of that, so thank you.

Kimberley Holt

From a doctor – Mum had come to the hospital with her new baby. He was gorgeous and about six days old. Mum's brother has DS and she had been given a low chance of DS on her screening. Several of her family members had said to her that her new baby looked like her brother when he was born and had openly asked her if the baby had DS. They had clearly worried Mum and Dad. Mum knew a lot about DS and was only worried because her brother had had a lot of cardiac problems and required multiple surgeries. She was asking me if her baby had DS.

I examined him. He at certain angles had some facial features of DS but no other features and my gut feeling was that he didn't have DS.

I had your voice ringing in my ears as I spoke to these new parents. I wanted to provide a balanced view but remain positive. We had a long chat and agreed that whether he had DS or not he was absolutely gorgeous and it really wouldn't matter either way. I was a bit of a wimp, however, and hedged my bets. I didn't say, 'I don't think your baby has DS' and went with something vague like I wasn't 'convinced'. Is that awful? It felt right at the time but afterwards felt like a poor choice of words (that's you getting in my head about this stuff again).

I asked a colleague to review but as they were busy and I wasn't a hundred per cent sure, and as the parents wanted something definitive I sent the blood test to look for DS.

I saw them again five days later and was sure that the baby didn't have DS when I looked at him, he was the spitting image of his mum. I still wasn't brave enough to say it until I went and collected the blood test results that confirmed the baby did not have any form of trisomy (the lab had tested for Edwards and Patau as well, despite me not asking for it). His parents were obviously relieved but it got me thinking about how the conversation would have gone had the bloods gone the other way. Would our talk from five days earlier haunt them in the same way that your paediatrician's 'Sorry' does you (I know haunt is the wrong word but can't think how else to put it)? Would I have said, 'Sorry'? Probably. How would I have broken the news? I was in the unusual position of having had a long chat about possible DS and what would happen from a medical perspective if he did have DS. I felt uncomfortable at the thought of having to tell them a DS diagnosis following on from our conversation last week. Now that's a strange thing to say; obviously there is always trepidation about giving someone any form of 'bad news', to use the medical education expression, but this was different. Was it because of the talk a few days earlier or was it because of your blog making me so much more aware of how any misspoken word will linger in that family's minds. I don't know. It's just how I felt.

Anyway, it's just a recent example of the many ways reading your blog has influenced me and how I speak to parents. Still love the blog and read regularly.

Anon

PS: Sorry about using the phrase 'features of DS'. I would never normally say that to a parent but medical language is so engrained in me that I can't explain what I mean in a better way here. I hope you don't take offence to it.

CHAPTER NINE

'Being a mother is learning about
strengths you didn't know you had and dealing
with fears you didn't know existed.'
– LINDA WOOTEN

People often ask me how I felt going from one child to two. Had I found it much harder work? Asking, if I had my time again, would I have such a small age gap or would I have waited a bit longer between the two? And, honestly, now that I'm in the throes of the carnage that *three* small children create (yes, after Alfie, I went on to have another, but more on that later), the appeal of just two kids sounds pretty wonderful right now. I don't doubt there was an adjustment back then though. I didn't have just Oscar to consider any more. I now had a newborn baby *and* a toddler – and, in what can only be described as perfect timing, Oscar had just started running around (did I mention that as soon as Oz started walking, he's literally never stopped?). But did Oscar and his DS bring further challenges to the table that a typically developing child wouldn't have? I'm not so sure. I'm wondering if things were any crazier than they would have been if I'd have had two without any additional needs.

I'm not denying that having Oscar has meant extra appointments. Whether they be health-related (heart, thyroid, hearing, etc.) or intervention-related (SALT – speech and language therapy; OT – occupational therapy: physio, etc.), having Oscar in our lives has meant we spend more time in hospitals, health centres and developmental play sessions. I always talk about the different level of care Oscar needs and how it takes longer to master stuff (I mean he's five right now and the toilet-training is still a work in progress) but has bringing Oscar up in day-to-day life differed that much from the other two? I'm not altogether sure it has. I mean, I suppose there were phases that lasted a bit longer. For example, although Oscar could manage his finger foods, he definitely wasn't spoon-feeding himself by this point. At mealtimes, when Alfie was weaned, for example, there was a lot of 'one for Oscar, one for Alfie' going on.

When I had Alfie, Oscar initially hadn't been walking. And even after he did, it took him a while to negotiate steps or uneven ground. Oscar, from the very beginning, has been a 'runner'. A term used among the DS community to describe a child who bolts. Runs off out of the blue, with no thought or consideration for the consequences of his or her actions. And that might be the same for any child of Oscar's age at this time but, like I say, the phase lasted a long old time – in fact, even now, on the odd occasion, if he decides he wants to make a dash for it, he'll still be off.

So, after Alfie was born and Oscar was up on his feet, I recall spending an awful lot of time chasing Oz while abandoning Alfie in his pram/car seat by the side of the road. One thing I often tell the parent of a child going on to have another post having a child with DS first, is to make sure you get a fabulous double-buggy. That you also need to find yourself a pair of trainers and don't *ever* take your eyes off the prize (the prize, metaphorically speaking, being Oscar).

Yep, that's probably the best bit of advice I can give to those people. Remember that children like Oscar can at times outrun you, outsmart you and leave you for dust. So never forget the unpredictability of your kids. Especially in a car park or wide open spaces.

In the early days, though, Alfie was a pretty chilled baby. My sister used to joke with me that he spent more time in his bouncy chair than any baby she knew. He did, because I guess like most people with toddlers, my attention was inevitably on Oscar. In fact, you'd often find Alfie in his chair, up on a table or the kitchen worktop, mainly because he was out of grabbing range of Oscar.

I always used to bath both boys together. Oscar had never been fazed by Alfie being in there. But I do remember this one time, after I repeatedly told Oscar not to grab Alfie's belly button, Oscar laughing and then going in for a bite of his tackle. Luckily, Alfie was rarely upset. Unless blood was drawn, of course (a different story today, when he'd most definitely give as good as he got). But I do remember around this time wondering if the 'terrible twos' were kicking in early (Oscar at this point was fast approaching his second birthday) or if this was the start of what I was to be faced with for years to come.

You see, even though I told myself not to google or look anything up, of course, I still did. I was still a member of a forum online, where parents like us could write about their recent experiences and worries and I could see how the future might be looking to us down the line. That pesky internet again. I guess I'd wanted to know what I might have to face later on and, at this stage, discipline had always been a big thing for me. I used to watch friends of mine when their children were playing up and I was in awe of the way they dealt with it … and then, sometimes, in a few cases, I watched and thought that perhaps I might have dealt with it differently because it didn't seem much like that they had control of the situation. Some, in my opinion, had it spot on, others (sorry friends) … not so much.

I naively watched shows like *Supernanny* way before I had Oscar and Alfie and thought how much sense it all made and how, when my turn came around, I'd totally have this nailed. But in reality, now that I was here faced with a toddler and a newborn, I wondered how the flippin' hell I was going to deal with it. I didn't have the first clue. How very different things are when you're not the one being Miss Judgey and it's actually you that's got to parent. So, apologies to all those friends and family members I silently judged.

I thought I knew what I wanted to do: I wanted to treat Oscar just as I would any other child, but there was something at the back of my mind back then questioning whether this was right. I wasn't sure if he fully understood, you see. He was still so young, right? I wondered if I should be giving him a little bit of a break, knowing that it might take him longer to compute things. But then, if I left it too late to try to educate him in what was right and wrong, wasn't there a danger the time would have passed, and I'd be one of those mothers on *Supernanny*, rocking in the corner, crying into her gin? I genuinely wasn't sure how to play it.

Of course, I knew that Oscar was far from stupid.

He understood a lot more than he let on. Was I confusing naughtiness with excitement in his newfound independence and exploration? All behaviours are a form of communication, I was once told. But was I just making excuses? I didn't want to be a weak parent because, when I saw weak parents, their children appeared to be out of control to me. And by this, I mean both people with typical children and those with children who have DS. One thing I was adamant about, was that I didn't want to be like that.

For the most part, Oscar was a lovely big brother. If Alfie cried, he would go straight over to him and look at him really closely in concern, then make sure I was coming over to check on him. Then sometimes he'd go over to Alfie when he was sat in his chair and try to take his dummy out of his mouth. Although not so great for Alfie, it was testament to the number of hours that Oscar and I had spent in speech and language sessions – posting things into letterboxes and taking puzzles out of boards. If anything, the skill and precision he was using to whip a dummy out of his baby brother's mouth actually should have been commended.

Not too dissimilar to the parents of other, typically developing, children, I had to keep a close eye on Oscar when he was around Alfie. He had a tendency to be rough with him at times and on a couple of occasions I found him on top of Alfie in the chair, having launched himself onto him, thinking it a game. He would stroke his head gently a few times but then go in for a dig of the nails, I think perhaps for attention or maybe to get a reaction. I mean, the sounds of Alfie's piercing cries were enough of a reaction for anyone. Crikey! Invariably, though, Oscar would have a little laugh at this and go on his merry way. Attention or reaction? Who knows?

One bit of advice I was given back then was by a SALT. She advised that you really shouldn't say 'No' at all to a child with DS. I understand the reason for this is that children who happen to have DS respond to positive reinforcement rather than negative, but I found it really hard. I know I tried to turn it round. So, instead of saying, 'Oscar, don't whack your brother with your new trainer' (he liked to carry his new Converse trainers around the house), I'd say, 'Gentle hands, Oscar.' I tried to praise all the good things he did, when he was kind and tried to help, but if he did hurt Alfie, I tried not to give him too much attention or focus on what he'd done. Instead, I would focus on Alfie, turning away from Oz, so that he understood he'd done wrong.

Around about this time I joined a group on Facebook, primarily for parents of children with DS. They mostly posted their achievements, their worries and concerns and it really was just an amazing support group to tap into, as and when I needed it. However, sometimes I read stuff that felt like I was looking just that little bit too far ahead. I always try to live in the present and not think about what hurdles we may have to face in years to come. But sometimes there was a voyeuristic side of the group that could make for tough reading. When Oscar was really little, I read a post from a mother of a six-year-old boy who also had DS. She talked openly of how she had gotten two black eyes because he'd lashed out at her. I remember reading it and feeling a wash of fear over me. What if Oscar was going to be like that? Would I/we be able to handle him? How would we be able to cope with that?

By the same token, though, I recall reading another post, by a mum of a little girl who was coming up for two years old, the same age as Oscar was at that time. The mum talked of how recently her girl had started lashing out, pulling hair and, I guessed, just generally testing boundaries. Oscar had been doing all of the above, too, and I'd wondered if it had been in direct response to having a new baby brother. Had it been typical behaviour of any eighteen-month-old or was this to be expected, because of the Down syndrome? One thing I did know was that there were so many responses from so many of the members, all of whom gave sound advice, which genuinely proved really helpful.

I think it took me a while to fully understand just how much of an impact Oscar having DS had on his development. I don't think I truly got it until I had my other two children and saw how quickly and easily they grasped things. How things that had taken Oscar months to master, the other two, on reflection, just did straight away.

In the past, Oscar has been described as naughty. I will never forget the time, as I was walking into his nursery to collect him one evening, a little girl was coming out and looked me square in the eye, turned to her Daddy beside her and said, 'That's naughty Oscar's mummy.' And I guess to another child or perhaps someone in the street who didn't fully understand, he may seem a little naughty.

When we used to be around children of the same age as Oscar, I would listen to their parents talk to them, asking them various questions, and I'd see recognition in their little faces. 'Do you want some more juice?' their mummies would ask and they'd either vocalise with a 'Yes, please' or nod their head. With Oscar, at this stage, if I'd had asked him, 'Do you want more juice?' he'd just look up at me smiling or stare blankly.

This is where Makaton, a language programme, came into play. From when he was a very young age, we were advised to start signing to Oscar to support our speech with him. Makaton is a form of sign language, although nowhere near as advanced or as complex as British Sign Language (BSL), but it is there as a visual cue for children like Oscar. Makaton uses signs and symbols to help people to communicate. It is designed to support spoken language and is deployed in spoken word order. Being able to communicate is one of the most important skills we need in life. Almost everything we do involves communication; everyday tasks such as learning at school, asking for food and drink, sorting out problems, making friends and having fun. These all rely on our ability to communicate with each other, so having this tool and developing it from an early age really helped us. Oscar was able to make himself understood, which obviously relieved a lot of frustrations. We started by signing things like 'more' and 'milk' and at times there were glimmers of recognition, but for Oscar it took a while.

There was a gorgeous little boy at Digbies (our support playgroup) who was about ten months older than Oscar. He seemed to understand a lot and I recall asking his mum at what point she realised that he was starting to know what she was saying. She said that I shouldn't underestimate just how much Oscar understood but that it would come over time – and she was so right.

I was told he would do some things that exasperated me and that was true and still stands true now. And while I know I might have to change my expectations of my child with additional needs to an extent, I have come to the conclusion that I don't have to lower my standards when it comes to wanting him to behave appropriately.

Sure, I knew it was going to take him longer to grasp things, but I still wanted him to conform as much as the next child. I guess it would have been easy to let my child who happens to have Down syndrome get away with behaviours you wouldn't tolerate in other children. But Oscar needed to know, early on, what I expected from him. Like all children, Oscar had to be taught to adjust to family routines and to manage himself, even if it might take a little longer. In much the same way, I had to learn patience.

I hoped others wouldn't make excuses for Oscar. People have a habit of struggling to deal with children who have DS and any behavioural issues they might have. They make excuses for them instead of telling them off. I guess we all need to think, what would we say to a 'typical' child if they were being naughty? None of this, 'Ah, bless him, he doesn't understand. Let him get away with it.' Maybe he hadn't quite grasped whatever it was *yet*, but if we were to let him get away with it now, there'll be problems ahead. By this time there had already been a few examples that had reaffirmed the fact that Oscar was definitely not stupid. In fact, he knew exactly what he was doing and would probably have been laughing at all those pitying him.

Around this time, Oscar was lucky enough to be accessing a service called portage. Portage is a home-visiting educational service for preschool-age children with SEND (Special Educational Needs and Disabilities) and Oscar's portage teacher was a lady called Sue. She came to our house regularly to help us develop skills in learning and playing together so that Oscar was able to participate and be included in his community in his own right. Both Oscar and I became very attached to Sue. I think she was one of the first professionals that gave me a bit of hope. She was enthusiastic about the future and the potential Oscar had, but mostly she understood some of the worries I had, too. I remember in one particular session, when Oscar was a little more excitable than normal, asking her if she thought this was an indicator that the future was going to be harder for us, discipline-wise. Her response was, 'Sarah, he's a little boy. He's almost two. Regardless of the Down syndrome, he's doing exactly what little boys of his age do.'

I recall back then always wanting to ask professionals what they thought. Do you think he's doing well? Do you think he'll ever walk? Ever talk? Get a job? My mind would race as I longed for their recognition of how well he was doing. But equally, if one of them said what I deemed to be a negative comment, I'd hold on to that and worry for days that he wasn't capable and was never going to amount to anything. I don't react so strongly as much now. Five years on, I think I'm learning to stop seeking praise and I'm simply just riding the waves with him. He has months where he'll be flying

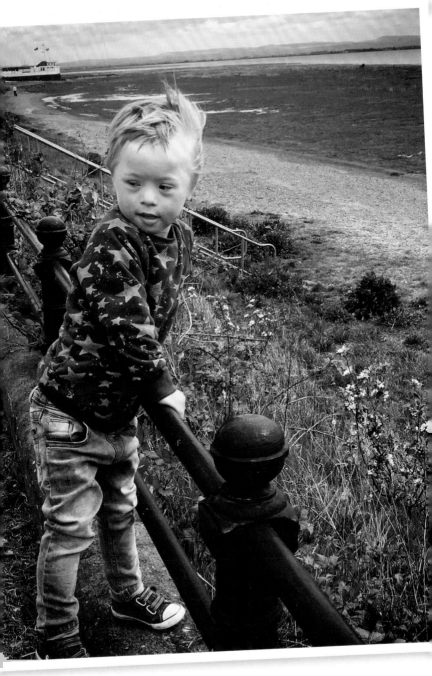

Oscar on the prom at Lytham St Anne's.

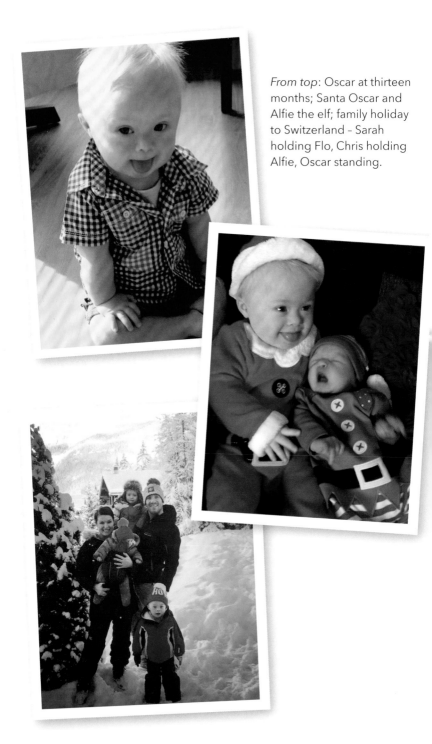

From top: Oscar at thirteen months; Santa Oscar and Alfie the elf; family holiday to Switzerland – Sarah holding Flo, Chris holding Alfie, Oscar standing.

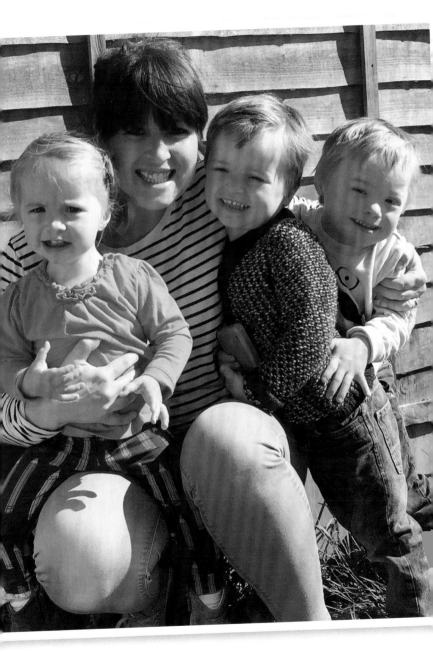

Mother's Day 2017.

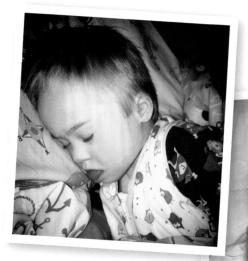

Clockwise from top left: Oscar asleep; after surgery for his ear cholesteatoma; Chris with the boys – too tired to walk . . .; out for a walk on the local common.

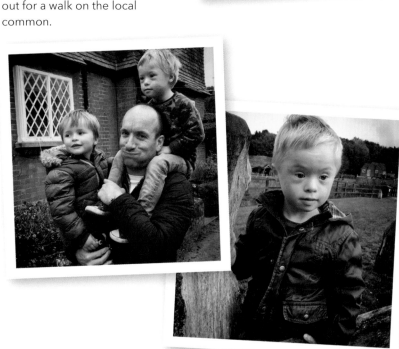

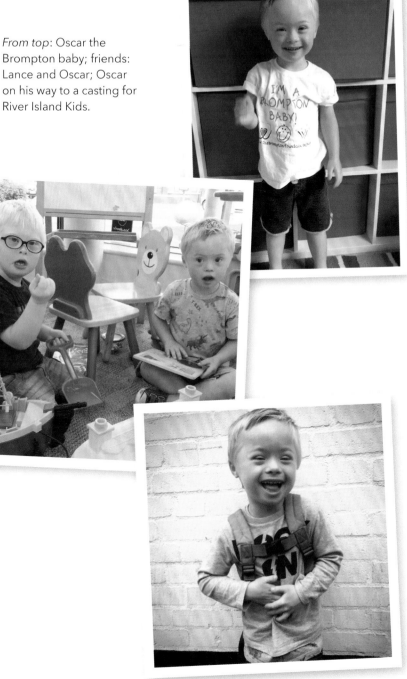

From top: Oscar the Brompton baby; friends: Lance and Oscar; Oscar on his way to a casting for River Island Kids.

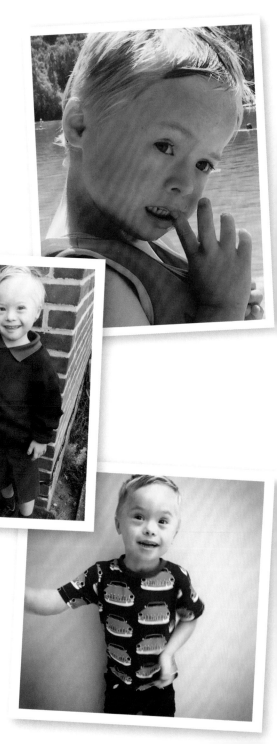

From top: Oscar on holiday; Alfie and Oz: brothers; modelling.

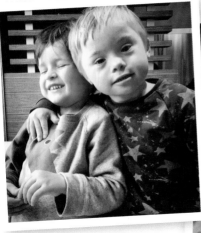

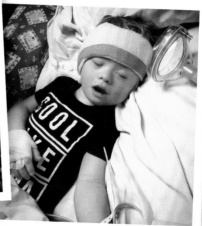

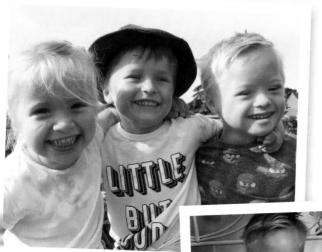

Top left: McDonald's time for Alfie and Oscar.

Top right: asleep after another surgery.

Middle: park life! with Flo, Alfie and Oz.

Bottom: Oscar's fifth birthday.

From top: Oz, Alfie and Flo crafting; bath time; Oscar's first day in Year 1 and Alfie's first day in Reception – September 2018.

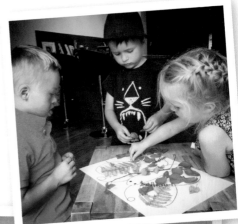

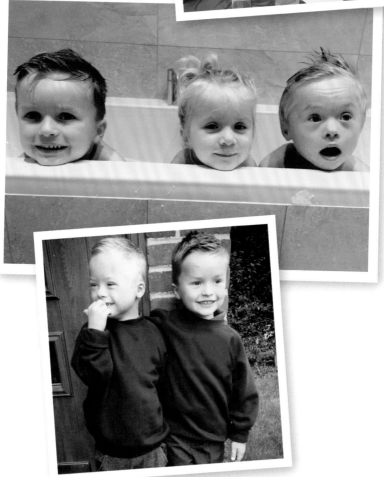

and others where I feel like he's stagnant or taking a step back. I think, though, it's easy for all of us to blame the DS. To put limitations on our kids just because of their label or diagnosis. It's easy for us to make excuses about what they are not achieving rather than celebrating all the things they are.

And when I was doing research on that pesky internet again, I came across something a mummy of a young boy who had Down syndrome had written. She said, 'Treat others how you would wish to be treated yourself and don't underestimate the ones "you think" don't understand ... because they more than likely do and they are more likely to be laughing at and pitying you, than you are them.' I hoped this was true of Oscar. With that mischievous smile that cropped up daily back then, I'm pretty sure he had us all sussed.

Blog comments

My sister is an adult (who happens to have Down syndrome). She lives with me and is a gift and an inspiration. She contributes around the house both with chores and laughter. Her emotional intelligence is immense – she challenges us to work out our problems and offers love and hugs when we need it. There are some responsibilities, things she needs help with, but that is rewarding.

It is a gift to be in that role. Sadly, people won't understand this if they haven't experienced it. And, as education and opportunity has advanced for these folks, their true capabilities are emerging. I see no reason that people with DS can't be independent and contribute to our society with their many gifts. We as a society need to stop limiting them by our low expectations of them.

Sonya Wachowski

Zach is the youngest of six. It does come down to love and strong family bonds. Our children love each other and we know they'll always be there for him. We have plans in place. When I voiced my concerns about Zach's well-being after we've passed and said how I didn't want him in care, my children actually got cross with me and told me that would never happen to their brother. Isn't it sad, though, that I was worried about the possibility of him being in care? Love my kids.

Elly Hardimou

CHAPTER TEN

*'Children have the unforgivable habit
of growing up.'*

– BJARNE REUTER, *THE RING OF THE
SLAVE PRINCE*, 2003

When Oscar turned two, he became eligible for fifteen hours a week of FEET funding (Free Early Education for Two-year-olds). We could use this in a nursery setting or with childminders. Sue had told us about this service as, funnily enough, the government don't come knocking at your door to let you know that you're entitled to it. Surprising, that!

In theory, it's the same as the fifteen hours (which has since been increased to thirty hours a week) that typically developing children are entitled to, only children with SEND receive it a whole year earlier.

I was keen for Oscar to start attending a nursery.

Aside from the fact that having some time with Alfie on my own would be great for the both of us, I knew that socially Oscar would love being around his peers. Chris and I were adamant at this point that we felt it was important for Oscar to attend a mainstream setting. We realised fairly early on that he loved other children and would often copy their behaviours. But picking a nursery didn't turn out to be straightforward, as there were a few settings out there which at first claimed they'd be happy taking a child with DS but the reality, when I went to visit them, was so very different.

You get a gut feeling when you're a mum, you see. In fact, I think you probably get more of a gut feeling about a lot of things when you've a child with SEND. You're their biggest advocate. So, when you visit a nursery setting and you can see the manager shifting nervously in her seat when you talk about your child, you kind of want to tell them where to stick their nursery place. If your child isn't going to be seen as an asset, if they don't believe that having them there would actually be really rather lovely, as opposed to a burden, there is no way in hell you're going to sign them up, right?

I recall how I felt before Oscar started at his new nursery. We had chosen it because it had not only come highly recommended by a couple of friends who already had children there but also I'd taken Oscar to have a look around and they couldn't have been more positive and welcoming. The staff had all been so engaging, the management unfazed by having him there – I mean, I'm sure they'd seen it as a challenge (for a start, there's a whole heap of extra paperwork that comes with having a child with SEND in your setting) but they didn't for one second ever see him as a burden on them.

I'd had mixed emotions in the run-up to him starting. I knew I felt confident with our decision but at the time there were so many worries whirling round my head. Would he be OK? Would he fit in? Would he be able to cope? Would they be able to cope with him? And I know that *every* mummy out there worries about their children, regardless of whether they have additional needs or not, but when I first enrolled Oscar I was adamant he should go somewhere that was all about inclusion and treating him just like any other two-year-old, but I remember panicking, once we'd said all that out loud, wondering if we were kidding ourselves. I don't think it was a question back then of me worrying that he wasn't capable. I knew he was doing really well and that at the age he was, he wouldn't necessarily need the one-to-one support he required as he'd gotten older, but I knew that there were some areas that he most definitely was going to need extra help with and I was mindful that I didn't want him to be seen as a pain before he'd even started.

I was apprehensive initially that Oscar was going to

be seen as the naughty kid. I doubt he was any more of a handful than the other two-year-old boys they'd had there, but I knew, as his mummy, he wasn't always the easiest of toddlers. Take, for example, when we'd go to a friend or family member's house. I would spend the first few minutes after we'd arrived doing a risk assessment on the place. You're probably thinking that this was so he didn't hurt himself. Um, no … it was more that he didn't end up breaking their stuff. I'd fear for the lives of lamps, ornaments – anything that he was not supposed to touch, and which he, without doubt, would have got his hands on. If it was up high, somehow he'd find it and get to it. He was a monkey. I'd find myself constantly saying, 'No' (even though I had that SALT's words ringing in my ears about 'positive reinforcement'). But even when I'd said 'No', it was probably only about 5 per cent of the time that he'd actually listen to me. He'd obviously inherited his dad's selective hearing (yep, Chris often filters out a lot of the things I say and probably only responds to a small percentage of it).

We'd had a meeting at Oscar's new nursery just before he was about to start. The SENCo (special educational needs coordinator), Oscar's new key worker, Chris and I were in attendance. His 'team' were also invited – his portage worker, his physio, a lady from hearing support as well as his early support worker. We'd all sat around and talked through any concerns we'd had. It definitely went well but I still came away feeling a bit sick. Chris, true to form, was completely confident.

'Do you think he'll be OK, Chris?' I'd said.

'Yeah, of course, Juts.' (Juts was his nickname for me. My maiden name had been Jutsum and apparently if you're from the north of England, as he is, the done thing is to abbreviate surnames. Who knew!)

'Yeah ... but do you think his key worker really "understands" Down syndrome?' I continued.

'She has a good heart and she loves Oz. He'll be fine.'

I remember worrying in the beginning about issues that I'd now consider so minor. The first was his drinking. All the other children had their own water bottles that the nursery had provided. Oscar had tried every beaker, sippy cup and bottle going and had only just mastered one that he could drink from himself without any help. They'd said that it would be fine for him to use his own, but as I'd watched the other children go over to get their water, I realised Oscar might not register what they were doing. He wasn't at the stage of asking for a drink so they were going to need to take it to him and offer it. And, just as I did, they were gonna have to persist until he drank some because, quite honestly, he could have taken or left it back then. He'd have been far too busy having fun to want a drink. So, yeah, the voice inside my head was saying they were going to find him a hindrance on day one.

I told his key worker that she was going to have to use short sentences or just key words or phrases with Oscar. It was important that she was clear and concise so as not to over-complicate things. Repeating words had been working for him and we talked about using visual aids, something he'd done in therapy and with me at home. I'd taken photos of his favourite things (his ball, his shoes, his milk, his toothbrush, his duck, etc.) and, thinking back, he'd really started to recognise the correct one when I'd offer him the choice. I had been encouraged to use photos and visual aids to help him in his new setting, especially at first. I thought perhaps they could have one for lunchtime, snack time, water break, circle time, nap time, etc. At least then he'd start to know what was required of him.

When I'd approached the nursery about this, all I could think were that they were thinking, OK – forget the kid, *how* annoying is his mother being with all these demands for extra equipment? I remember explaining that although he was more than capable of putting a toy down after he was finished with it, occasionally he'd throw it. There was a reason for this. I had found out that it apparently takes far more effort and energy for children who happen to have DS to place a toy down, using the release motion, than it does to cast it away. I worried that Oz would be chucking stuff left, right and centre. That staff and children would be dodging Duplo bricks and various cuddly toys as they flew through the air. I also said that sometimes it was a very deliberate cast and if that was the case, then by all means they should please call him up on it.

One of my biggest concerns before he started nursery was what would happen if he was struggling with whatever activity the rest of the group were doing. I worried that staff would sit him down in a corner and occupy him with something else, not allowing him to partake in what everyone else was doing because it'd be too much effort to involve him. My biggest fear was that he wouldn't meet his full potential in a mainstream setting because people might baby him or wouldn't give him the time he needed. But I'd also worried that a specialist school wouldn't push him enough, so who really knew what the answer was? I just desperately didn't want them to leave my Oscar out. I worried that they wouldn't take him outside if that's where everyone else was going. I worried they'd assume he'd follow. I worried that it was more than likely that he'd actually decide he'd much rather empty all the bricks on the floor for no apparent reason or saunter over to the paints and start wandering around with the brushes in the air, bumping into a doorframe as he went because he'd be too engrossed in whatever he'd been doing to actually notice everyone else had gone out. I wanted to shout, 'He *loves* being outside but he won't necessarily realise that's where you're all going, so please take him because he'll have the best time out there!' I was probably doing him a disservice. At home, he totally knew when the back door was open, or any door anywhere, for that matter. He'd dart out quicker than a flash, so who was I kidding? He'd figure it out soon enough.

They'd asked in this meeting about behaviour. For the most part, I actually think at this stage Oscar was pretty good. Aside from the initial whirlwind he created when he entered somewhere new, he was usually quite happy playing and amusing himself. I recall though they asked if he pushed and I said, no, he'd only push if someone was in his face and if he did, it'd never be out of malice. They then asked about biting, which at the time of the meeting he didn't do but, of course, just to add to my anxiety levels, he started biting shortly after he started.

While we were in the meeting, Oscar spent some time in the nursery and, to put us parents at ease, they had had the CCTV display in our meeting room so we could watch his every move on the monitor. As it happened, I had my back to the screen so couldn't see what was going on, but throughout the meeting, every once in a while, I'd catch Chris looking up at the screen and smiling. He told me on the way home that Oscar couldn't have timed things better. When they were asking if Oscar pushed, there was me saying, 'No,' then with that, two little boys came over to him and he pushed them both away. When

I was talking of my concerns about casting, he threw a toy across the room and the nursery staff member had to come over to pass it back to him. Finally, when they asked what his general behaviour was like and I was saying pretty good, at that moment Oscar was climbing to get on the table. Chris found all this hilarious; I, on the other hand, felt a wave of panic rush over me.

I had been torn back then, you see ... on the one hand, I was worrying about leaving them with my baby, my first-born who, let's face it, was going to need a watchful eye. On the flip side, I was worrying that my little pickle would cause complete and utter havoc. Yet I knew he'd be OK. I knew he'd love it, he'd thrive and probably wouldn't even look back to say 'Goodbye'.

Someone once said that 'love is learning to let go'. Relinquishing the control and trusting your child into the arms of someone else had to happen sometime and I knew that that in doing so, I was doing the right thing by Oscar. If you truly love someone, you set them free if they want to go. I had to allow him to go but, my god, did it hurt. I'd hoped back then that my fears would be squashed once he'd started and that Oscar's transition into the nursery would be a success. I'd hoped that the nursery staff had patience and understanding and could appreciate that with a little extra attention, there would be no limits to what Oscar could achieve. I'd hoped that Oscar himself proved my fears wrong, behaved beautifully and didn't cause too much trouble. I was confident that regardless of any tables he might climb on or toys he might throw, he would charm them with that face of his and they would fall in love him, like we all have.

And once he started, that's what happened. All my fears were squashed, of course. Don't get me wrong, he did, at times, cause trouble. There were the odd behavioural issues here and there (like the time he got hold of the black paint and painted one of the hallways with it, or the time he bit the same girl four times in one day) but from the very beginning the nursery embraced Oscar. They engaged with him, they understood the concepts of inclusion and integration and did everything they could to make his time there the best is could possibly be.

When I'd had Oscar, I didn't allow myself to think too far ahead. The future was a scary place and allowing myself to wonder how life would be, even in a couple of years' time, was sometimes too much. But here he was, two years on, living a pretty lovely life. He was, I was happy to admit, a million and one miles away from where I'd first imagined he might be.

Blog comments

On 1 September 2015, I posted a photo of Oscar and I leaving for nursery. I wrote: 'After three settling-in sessions of a few hours here and there, today was Oscar's first official full day at nursery.

'I am told he did brilliantly, eating most of his lunch and tea (apparently including six mini-tuna and cheese sandwiches. Yes, six!). He had a go at body painting but wasn't the biggest fan of paint between his toes. Danced along to all the songs but was particularly partial to "Old MacDonald" and when I arrived was happily playing with the musical instruments! He even had a nap on a mat on the floor! I am amazed!

'So all in all a great success! Long may it last, Oz.'

That's awesome, Sarah! Mikey had his first day at nursery today, too! He also slept on a mat on the floor and I too was amazed. These boys of ours always surprise us, hey?

Stacey Sampson

So cute! Kids are great in nurseries as they copy their peers! I struggle to get Poppy to sit through a whole meal at home, but she's perfect at pre-school! Bet you cried today, though.

Lianne Brinklow

Bet you were on pins all day, and there was
nothing to worry about. Good old Oscar.

Margaret Jarman

Well done, li'l fella. Gracie just started two weeks
ago as well. It's such a worry, isn't it! I think we
worry far more than we need to!

Anon

CHAPTER ELEVEN

'People see what they want to see and what people want to see never has anything to do with the truth.'
– ROBERTO BOLAÑO, CHILEAN NOVELIST

I come from a family of three girls. I was the oldest and then had two younger sisters. We lived in a small village in the country and every Sunday our parents would take us to church. This is going to make us sound like we were deeply religious. I don't think we were especially.

I think perhaps it was more about instilling good values into us as children and that was why Mum and Dad took us along each week. I know they also liked the sense of community the church brought us, which in hindsight I think was really rather lovely. From what I remember, everyone in our village knew everyone else. I recall a lot of things about church – playing Mary in the

Nativity and having to ride in on one of the bigger boy's backs (he was the donkey, obviously). My little sister Clare, who in the same Nativity was playing the part of one of the sheep, spent the entire time fidgeting and getting told off. I remember the uplifting songs, the man with the guitar, the fact that we got to leave halfway through the sermon to go and do arts and crafts and have a biscuit, but my standout memory was of a girl. The girl I'm thinking of must have been five or six years older than me. I remember her wearing thick brown boots all year round, how she walked strangely and didn't really say much. When she did I remember thinking that I didn't understand her and I also remember her doing some weird shouting at the top of her voice from time to time. I was intrigued by her. I'd found her fascinating, but I also remember so vividly how scared I was of her.

I often think back to this girl now as I'm well aware that the reason I felt frightened was that I'd never been around anyone like her. She wasn't like the other children who came to church. Sure, you could talk to her but you wouldn't get anything back. It was so obviously apparent that she was different.

When I think about Oscar and the way he's been treated over the years, I genuinely feel, for the most part, that he has been met by positivity and understanding. I think that because he looks the way he does – in that he obviously looks like he has Down syndrome – people are perhaps more open to him and his idiosyncrasies. From time to time, people will stare or we might get the odd remark but, mostly – because I think we, as a society, are so much more inclusive of 'different' – he is very much accepted.

I think children in society today are perhaps that bit further ahead than the previous generation. They're more accepting of 'different' because in their playgroups, schools, dance classes etc., there are many different children, whether it be race, ethnicity, religion, sexuality or disability. Back when I went to school and in our white, very middle-class village, there was perhaps one other pupil in our school of 'different' origin. But, certainly, no one who had a disability. We were all very much deemed the same.

By the same token, children can often say what they see. There is no filter. They just say it. We are no stranger to comments about Oscar such as, 'Why does his tongue stick out like that?' or, 'But why can't he talk?' When I explain to them that Oscar can say some words but that he struggles with his speech and he's just going to take that extra bit of time to learn, they'll often look at me, think about it for a second and shrug it off as no big deal. I love kids for that.

Oscar coped so brilliantly with his transition into nursery. He never appeared fazed that I was leaving him there for extended amounts of time and always seemed genuinely pleased when we'd pull into the car park. But after a short time, his 'biting' phase seemed to crank up a level. By this time he was around two and a half. He'd adapted well to having a baby brother around and had, thankfully, stopped smacking Alfie on the forehead, making him topple over when sitting up or attempting to walk. I was grateful he was out of that phase, but the biting thing, for me at the time, I really struggled with. I can look back now and think, 'Hey, he was only two and half. A lot of young children do that sort of thing, regardless of having a learning disability.' But Oscar's biting phase went on and on and got to the point where I became anxious when taking him out anywhere.

I should mention again here that when Oscar was born, he had failed his initial hearing test and I wonder now if this led to a series of events that might have contributed to his biting. Shortly after the test he was diagnosed with glue ear. This is caused by congestion and it is fairly common in little ones with DS. The resulting hearing loss was mild to moderate and that meant it was not a major physical problem and could potentially clear as he got older. But the thing that worried me was the effect on his mental development – these early years were crucial and if he couldn't hear properly, our concern was that he would have trouble picking up speech. It was decided that we should fit him with a BAHA (bone-anchored hearing aid). These hearing aids are the type that are fixed on a band and sit on the bone behind his ear. They work by sending vibrations through the bone so that sounds are magnified for the wearer.

From the start, I hated it. I mean, I had a real bee in my bonnet about it. Had this kid not had enough to deal with? And now he was being expected to look like some eighties throwback rocker with a god-awful headband. Oscar wouldn't tolerate it either. He repeatedly tore it off and threw it away. If he was at the top of the slide, he loved nothing better than lobbing the headband from a great height, just for shits and giggles. We broke a lot – the hospital wasn't our biggest fan, I'm sure. But he was still only two and a half years old. He'd already shown an unwillingness to wear a sunhat in good weather and that hadn't instilled me with a huge amount of confidence that he was going to tolerate the hearing aid for any amount of time.

Since then, it has turned out that his hearing issues have been ongoing and he has had major problems. This takes us back to the biting. I can't say for sure that it was as a result of his struggles with hearing. Yet, even at the time of writing this, when he's just over five, if ever he's suffering with his ears, he can bite the odd child. I sometimes feel like that mum who makes excuses for her child, 'Oh, he didn't mean to bite your daughter. He's just brewing an ear infection I think,' blah, blah, blah. I'm sure others think that I'm just trying to cover for him but he's not a malicious kid and I think that it's just because he's uncomfortable, or maybe that it feels nice to bite down, that it still comes out from time to time (Chris has nicknamed him 'Jaws').

Anyway, this was the bane of my life. I'd be anxious about going to friends' houses, worried that he'd bite their kids. I'd never actually get to spend any time with the adults when we did go visiting; I was constantly having to shadow Oz in case he lashed out. Because here's the thing: nobody wants to be the parent who you think others are thinking badly of. If Oscar did bite someone, the chances are the parent of that other child, although understanding for the most part, would subconsciously be thinking, Well, where the bloody hell were you when it happened? Because I think I probably would if someone bit my child. Saying, 'Oh, I was having a cuppa with my mate in their kitchen, while my child was running ragged,' probably doesn't go down too well, funnily enough.

Anywhere where Oz felt restricted – e.g. in a Wendy house that he couldn't get out of because other children were in the way – he didn't have the communication skills to say, 'Um, excuse me, I need to get out.' Instead, he might bite the other child on the arm. If another child went in for a hug and he wasn't ready, he might feel too smothered and give them a nip. If he was on a bouncy castle (and still, if ever he's on one, even now,

I still hold my breath the entire time, my shoes off, ready to pounce) and someone fell on him or initiated rough-and-tumble, he was sure to bite. I also recall that back then when another child had a toy he'd wanted – again because he didn't have the language to say that he'd like a turn – on occasion he'd just go on over and bite them. He wasn't stupid, of course. He knew when we were watching him. And if we were, he didn't do it. Of course, as I write this, he very rarely bites. It'll only be once in a while and usually because he has an ear infection brewing and he doesn't really know what to do with himself. So I guess he has grown out of it – but as to whether it was a phase, down to his difficulty in communicating, or the fact that he had reoccurring ear problems for most of his toddler and preschool years and his early years at school life, who knows?

What I do know is that it was a difficult time. I think mainly because there's so many clichés about children with disabilities. Certainly, young children who have DS. Lots of people label them as being 'naughty' but I genuinely think that their behaviours are in direct response to wanting to be understood. It's just that it's hard for other people, adults and children, to see what's really going on. And that's the thing, isn't it? To other children, when kids like Oscar bite, lash out, climb on tables and take toys off them, that simply constitutes being naughty. That other child's not going to understand that the way that someone else behaves is because they have trouble communicating. They're perhaps going to think they're a little arsehole.

My worry though, was would people feel anxious about their children being around Oscar, knowing that he was capable of hurting another child? Would those people, my friends, decide they didn't want to have him in their friendship group, for fear that he might hurt their little ones? I am aware that I have a habit of being over-emotional at times and can also overthink things, but I couldn't shake the worry that others might feel this way. I guess I knew that children of Oscar's age, regardless of having additional needs or not, still constantly pushed one another, shouted at each other, fought over toys and so on, but maybe in a few years' time, when their children were fully aware of the consequences of their actions and Oscar was potentially still not quite getting it, would they then turn around and say, 'We've had enough of him'? I guess that was my biggest fear in all this. Were people not going to want Oscar in their lives?

I appreciated that when I thought back to my reaction to the girl in my church, that I had to remember that I was young. But what if Oscar's peers felt nervous around him? Even into my own teens and early adulthood, having not really been exposed to people with DS and having very little knowledge and understanding, I made a judgement. I gave my friends and family full credit and

I knew that they had lived life long enough not to be so narrow-minded and prejudiced as I once was, but if they were, could I blame them?

I recalled a friend of mine telling me that among another group of her friends, one of the children started biting. It turns out that one of the parents felt they couldn't let their child be at risk of being bitten, so sent an email to the mother, saying that she felt she could no longer mix in the same group. Hearing this, I felt sad. Because surely at some point every child goes through some kind of phase and although not every child bites, there are many other ways they can vent their frustrations. I was hoping with Oscar that people understood. And I'm hoping that anyone reading this that knows Oscar and me, knows that I did everything in my power to make it stop. To help him understand it wasn't acceptable and couldn't go on. I was hoping that people will give him a little bit of a break and give him that time. And I was so hoping that he/we would not lose friends over this.

Just recently we had some work done on our house. Nothing major, just some carpentry and decorating, but it meant that we had tradesman coming in and out. I knew very little about the gentleman who did the majority of the work, except that on first meeting he seemed a fairly quiet, unassuming but kind man. Over the course of the time he was with us, we gradually spoke a little more. He'd asked me in the beginning how old Oscar was and when I told him he just nodded and I could tell he was taking it all in. Following that brief exchange we got talking about Down syndrome and he volunteered, 'Before I came to work for you, I don't think I'd ever really met anyone with Down syndrome before.' He then went on to say that prior to meeting Oscar he knew he would have been cautious and kept his distance, 'not really sure how to act around him'. He said that since spending time around our family and seeing the way Oscar interacted with us, he'd realised that he should never have felt that way. He said that even though Oscar didn't say that much, he could see what a lovely personality he had and how engaged and switched-on he was. The workman said he spoke to his own sister and told her about us and she asked how we knew what Oscar wanted if he couldn't say it verbally and this man told me he'd said, 'It's amazing, they just do.'

I smiled as I walked away from our conversation. For I realised, without either Oscar or the man working for us realising it, my boy had educated him simply by being him. It's small on the grand scheme of things. I'm not saying one man's changed opinion or mindset is going to change the world, but it's about gently educating right?

I wouldn't like to say how old this gentleman was, but if I were to hazard a guess I'd say in his fifties. So even if it's taken him this long to have his eyes opened and his heart filled with someone like Oscar, well, that makes me very happy.

Blog comments

Hello! You don't know me, but I love reading your posts and seeing your dear children. I have four children – three neuro-typical and one less so. She has had many health, social and developmental issues over the years, many of which are resolved/ resolving, and I know what a privileged position that puts us in. Anyway, the reason I am messaging you is because I wanted to tell you what an amazing difference tonsil and adenoid removal made for our daughter. She didn't have visible tonsils (really not at all) and she had airflow through her nose, but she had awful asthma and regular pneumonias requiring admission to hospital as well as other issues. One amazing doctor, out of the blue, suggested a sleep study, and they found she was having multiple cessations of breathing throughout the night. This meant they recommended her immediately for tonsil and adenoid removal, and I can only say that it has completely transformed her life, our lives, her health, etc.

Fewer chest infections, a bigger, louder voice

(not necessarily an advantage!) and a patent airway
all night. It really has been a total game changer.
Her consultant says her tonsils were like *Titanic*
icebergs – only the tiny tip of them was showing,
but actually they were taking up a huge amount of
her poor airway.

Anon

I just wanted to share my story with you. I didn't
want to put it publicly for fear of what people
might say but I think it's really important that you
know what a difference your blog makes. Eighteen
years ago I found I was pregnant, I had various
scans and checks as usual and was referred for
additional tests. I was told at my local hospital
that my child had DS and was immediately given
literature on termination. I was a very innocent
twenty-two year old, unmarried and didn't have a
clue what DS was or the implications of it.

I was admitted to hospital with severe morning
sickness and bleeding around about six months'
pregnant and I think, in a way, I hoped that nature
would take its course. I was so very scared. I spoke
to a really wonderful doctor one evening and
he said to me that, no matter what, I shouldn't
consider a termination, he said he knew he
shouldn't advise me one way or another but he said

that each child was a blessing and that a child with DS was just like any other child, that they could go on to have the same lives that any other child had. He really touched a chord and I refused all further interventions once I was discharged from hospital.

My daughter Gaby was born in December 1999. She is now 17, she was born in a room full of medical teams and machinery and after full checks it turned out that she had been incorrectly thought to have DS due to other medical conditions. I often look at your photos and your site and feel really very thankful for it. I also have a tinge of guilt that I ever considered wanting to be without my own baby due to my own fears. I think your blog is amazing, it gives the advice that I really needed over seventeen years ago and I'm sure must be helping other scared prospective parents. So, thank you, I know you are all making a huge difference.

Anon

Hi, I just wanted to say thank you. We had a daughter called Sophie in May, she had Down syndrome but also quite a complex heart condition. She ended up having five open-heart surgeries and, after a long fight in the ICU over Christmas, she passed away at the end of January. We are obviously devastated, but I'm so glad to have had a baby with Down syndrome. Sophie was one of a kind; she was actually the best baby ever. This time last year I was terrified after receiving our diagnosis, but your blog (and the messages you sent) were some of the first things that calmed those fears and made me realise I didn't need to be sorry and people didn't need to be sorry for me. We've had the year from hell but I would absolutely do it over and over again to have that time with our girl and I wouldn't swap that Down syndrome for anything. I think we will go on to have other children in time, and I know that my first reaction if we are told that our baby doesn't have Down syndrome will be devastation! I can't imagine loving another baby as much as I love Sophie! Her Down syndrome made her that bit more than perfect. But I'm assured by many people I will love another kid anyway, ha! Anyway, thank you for the work you are doing to advocate on behalf of our kids. I hope to be able to do the same even though Sophie is no longer here. I always tell people about your blog. You are doing an amazing job.

Katie Garden

CHAPTER TWELVE

'When a flower doesn't bloom you fix the environment in which it grows, not the flower.'
– ALEXANDER DEN HEIJER

Oscar was *still* going through his biting stage (yeah, he stopped for about five weeks, lured me into a false sense of security ... but then started again – sigh) and that was causing me a lot of stress. My wobbles were increased when I was advised (and this was some advice I greatly appreciated, I might add) that I read a book called *The Out-of-Sync Child* by Carol Stock Kranowitz, as it might help me 'understand' Oscar.

I'll start at the beginning. Oscar, Alfie and I went on a trip to the supermarket, all in good spirits. I put Oscar and Alfie in the trolley but as soon as we set foot inside the supermarket, Oscar cried. When I say cried, I don't mean uncontrollably, it was more a moan of sorts. When he's upset he puts his finger in his mouth and chews down on it. It's something he's done since he was a baby and people often comment that he's teething when actually, he does it when he's upset or unsettled.

Presuming I was hearing a bit of a protest at him being cooped up in the trolley and not wanting to pander to him, I carried on with the job in hand. Knowing Oscar as I do, I thought he'd stop the waterworks soon enough. He's usually such a happy little boy (there's that annoying cliché that every parent of a child with DS hates) but in Oscar's case, for the most part, he really is! I was sure he'd stop, but he didn't. I tried everything. A drink, a snack, letting him play with my phone (I was desperate), singing, dancing down the aisles (me, not him, obvs), you name it, I tried it, but he was having none of it. After a long and stressful supermarket shop (I'm pretty sure this persuaded me to do my grocery shopping online from then on), we left, only for him to stop his moaning/protesting the very the second we exited the building. I expected him to be unwell later that day, or miserable, but he wasn't. He was as happy as Larry. I put this to the back of my mind, for a while at least.

The next day we had a consultation day at our local support group with some of Oscar's therapists. Every Friday we met with Oscar's peers, all of whom have DS, and the children go from room to room, doing their different therapies. There's OT, speech therapy and early years teaching and, of course, between the groups the parents get to chat while the children play. On the first week back in every term, the therapists talk to the parents about their child's progress, areas of concern and what's next for them. It was when I went in to see Oscar's speech therapist that things started to become a little clearer.

We agreed Oscar had made great progress, that we should continue working the way we had been and, although his concentration wasn't the best, it had absolutely improved. I felt happy that she had been so positive. She was an amazing therapist and we were so lucky to have her. But I had one thing on my mind that I had wanted to address. When Oscar's concentration wavered during the session, I had noticed that the therapist would often give him a chewy or buzzy, which he immediately brought to his mouth. He would start chewing down or would start to feel the vibrations of the buzzy that came through his mouth. I knew that, for whatever reason, it worked and that invariably, the distraction was all he needed to continue with the session and in my naivety, I asked why.

She started to explain that Oscar was a 'sensory seeker'. She was explaining as if I already knew this. And indeed, everything she was saying I agreed with – it was just that I hadn't realised there was an actual label for it or indeed an explanation. She said that sensory seekers simply can't get enough of any sensation, literally. And that anyone who suffers from the disorder (ouch, I hate that word) are constantly in search of ways to arouse their nervous system. She likened it to someone who might feel the need to incessantly tap their foot. It could be a comfort thing or a concentration thing, but if we were to feel an urge that needs to be satisfied, we work out that foot-tapping is what we need to do to remain calm and grounded. The difference is that a sensory seeker like Oscar might also be feeling a bit odd, but he can't work out what he needs to satisfy that.

She also explained that sensory seeking is a subtype of Sensory Processing Disorder (SPD) and that there were many different types of SPD. Oscar's variant could have manifested itself in the reverse way, in that he might have shied away from sounds, touch, smells, tastes. Instead, he sought them out. When I told her about the supermarket, she said it could have been any number of things bothering him, from the lights to the temperature and the background noise – things that perhaps weren't noticeable to me because I have learnt how to deal with those changes in my environment.

So here was where the book came in. And, while being so grateful that she was helping me understand, I couldn't help that wobbly feeling. I needed to read a book with a title like *The Out-of-Sync Child*. I mean, could it sound any more ... depressing?

While waiting for my Amazon book order to arrive, I took to Google. I know – you're thinking that I have already advised you not to google anything. It's the devil. And not only when it comes to DS. If you have a headache, you think it's a tumour. If you have a child that doesn't sleep, there are literally ten million reasons to help them (and no quick-fix guide to which one is the best solution for you), and if you have a child with DS and you google it, well, it can be the bleakest, most depressing thing in the world, according to what search results you return. Every once in a while though, Google is your friend. And in this, reading up on sensory seeking, Google helped me see things a lot more clearly.

It was literally like reading a blow-by-blow account of Oscar. I won't list everything that came back. There were a lot. But these in particular jumped out at me from the screen:

1. Loves loud noises, often watches TV and listens to music very loudly. (This *is* Oscar. He loves anything with the volume turned up or any toy that makes noises. He loves the traffic lights when they beep and an ambulance whizzing by with the sirens . He claps his hands, shouts and just generally gets excited at all of the above.)

2. May frequently make noises just to hear them. (A friend has a fireguard that makes a lovely

loud noise when you shake it. This was a great source of amusement for Oscar and even though I repeatedly took him away from the guard, he was drawn to it all afternoon.)

3. Will put anything in their mouth in search of oral input, such as chewing or crunching sensations – (He loves crisps for this reason I'm sure, and his latest, pomegranate seeds. I'm sure this is because they crunch in his mouth.)

4. May love or crave bright lights. (Always has done.)

5. May love to spin in circles. (When he does spin, which is not all the time, he'll often repeat it as he clearly loves the sensation of dizziness.)

6. Fidgets, has difficulty sitting still at times and takes bold risks. (Oscar to a T.)

7. May frequently jump from high heights. (Um … this is definitely him. He has no sense of fear but will often repeatedly jump from the arm of the sofa, rolling into the chair, then roll to the floor, like some kind of stuntman. But rest assured, we do *try* to stop this behaviour. It's an ongoing battle.)

8. May repeat certain movements almost endlessly just for the sensation. (See above – sigh.)

9. Frequently overstuff their mouth when eating. (He has done this from a young age, although

he's much better now. When I sign 'wait', for example, he'll make sure he does just that before he stuffs the next grape or McDonald's chip in his mouth.)

10. Problems sleeping. (Although not awful, and I mustn't complain because I know it could be a lot worse, he can have periods of time where he'll be wakeful throughout the night.)

11. Frequently attempts to engage in rough play, such as wrestling. (Tick – although so does Alfie, Daddy and Grumps, Oscar's grandad, so you can't really blame him.)

12. High levels of energy (He. Does. Not. Stop. Moving. All. Day!)

I knew that in the grand scheme of things this wasn't a major deal. It's just something that Oscar, Chris and I were going to have to try to manage and understand. His speech therapist told me she knew a little boy who had a different form of learning difficulty and that from the age of five, had hated PE at school. It wasn't until he was nine that he could articulate to her that it wasn't because he hated games and exercise, it was that he didn't like the way his feet felt in his plimsolls. I guess this just made me feel sad. Would Oscar be like this? Would he not be able to find the words to tell me what was bothering him in the future? Frustrations in communication come hand-in-hand with having a not-quite-three-year-old, but as he got older and might not be able to let me know was troubling him, there lay the problem that could contribute to behavioural difficulties.

I figured that all we could do was watch and learn. What were his triggers? Why was he acting the way he was and was he just being a typical little boy, or, as in the supermarket, was there something upsetting his balance? I read that there were treatments to explore – for example, putting him on a sensory diet or doing therapeutic listening, so in time I decided to take a look. I will say that finally understanding the reasons for some of the differences we had noticed in him was both a huge blessing and a relief. The whole thing was fascinating and perhaps my slightly dramatic hormonal state at that moment was kinda adding to my anxiety about it.

As a parent, you can spend hours on end worrying about your child – the truth of the matter is, he's Oscar, regardless of any label or diagnosis he's given. He's our little boy, who is loved more than ever and will continue to do brilliantly because simply, that is what he does by just by being him.

Blog comments

I'm pregnant now after Sophie. We went for the NIPT test. I took that because we definitely wanted to know beforehand so that I could be prepared for what might be in store, and also because I knew I was going to have to come to terms with this baby not having Down's and essentially not being Sophie. To be honest, I had a little cry when I got my letter back saying my 'risk' of having another baby with Down's was really low!! Obviously, it's good that the chances of extra health problems are much lower, but there's definitely a Down syndrome-shaped hole in my life! We were offered an amnio at about seven weeks which upset me a bit because I pretty much knew that the only reason they were offering it was so that if I wanted to terminate because of Downs I could do so sooner rather than later. My other reason for having the NIPT was that if I had it and the results came back as the baby having Down's and I kept the baby, then I was contributing to reducing the percentage of prenatal diagnoses that result in terminations, if that makes sense!

Katie Garden

Lucas (DS) is three and Jake (non-DS) is three months. Initially, the thought crossed my mind that I may have another with DS and would I cope with two disabled children? But by choice we decided not to have any tests; for us it was the right decision. We decided if our second was to also have DS it wouldn't change anything and we didn't want any doctors to try to influence our pregnancy like they did with our first. Doctors did not understand why we had opted for no testing but we stayed strong even though it was mentioned a lot. When Jake was handed to me I did not once think about whether he had DS or not – it just didn't come into my mind once.

Jasmine Corner

CHAPTER THIRTEEN

*'Education is learning what you didn't even
know you didn't know.'*

– DANIEL J. BOORSTIN, 'A CASE OF HYPOCHONDRIA',
NEWSWEEK, 6 JULY 1970

I haven't talked much about my blog and social media channels but, having started writing in 2014 and posting my first blog post on my own page, my following over the years has grown. I first started writing as an outlet. It was somewhere for me to record my thoughts and feelings and make sense of things. I'd never written anything before. OK, I tell a lie, I won a poetry competition they'd run in my local newspaper. But I was seven. And I don't think writing a poem about aliens would get me that much kudos these days.

As I mentioned earlier in the book, I remember the day I posted my first blog post on my personal Facebook page. Within a few hours it had had hundreds of shares. I guess those friends and family who had been following me on Facebook had wanted to pass it on. Someone suggested I create a public page which I did a few days later and the rest, as they say, is history.

To start with the blogs were only really about helping me make sense of how I was feeling, but I soon saw that after I had shared my story, others would come forward and tell me how much it was helping them. People had gone through similar experiences, whether it be that they'd had babies with DS themselves or perhaps had found out a bit later down the line that their child had had a different diagnosis – ASD (autism spectrum disorder), ADHD (attention deficit hyperactivity disorder), GDD (global development delay), etc. I soon realised that by writing stuff down and telling my truth, it was somehow helping others. In the first year of my writing, I won a MAD (Mum And Dad) Blog award for best new blog, which helped massively with my confidence. I couldn't believe that people had actually wanted to hear what I had to say but for some reason they did and from thereon, the blog has grown.

I now spend a great deal of my time giving talks in hospitals to healthcare professionals, highlighting the importance of the use of their language. I talk about how when we'd had Oscar and the paediatrician had uttered those words, 'I'm so sorry', her projecting to us that having Oscar and him having DS was the worst news imaginable. I explain how I felt so passionately about the fact that 'sorry' was quite possibly one of the worst things they could have said. Why did she have to start her sentence that way? Why hadn't she said, 'Congratulations, your son's beautiful'? Why didn't she just say, 'Listen, I know what I'm about to tell you won't be the news you were expecting but please don't panic, it really is going to be OK'? Why, in her position, as someone I respect and admire and whose opinion I so value, did she have to look so forlorn? This hadn't been the news we had expected, she would have been right about that, but that paediatrician's outlook was far removed from the actual reality of having Oscar. I still wonder now if she even spent five minutes with my boy, would her opinion change? Would she still be 'sorry'?

So many women and men contact me through my blog to tell me about the negative way the news that their baby had DS is delivered. So many feel strongly about the fact that it didn't need to be that way. I wonder if the day will ever come where people's perceptions will change and having a baby with DS won't be seen as being the end of the world?

As it stands at the moment here in the UK, you are legally allowed to have an abortion up until twenty-four weeks. However, if you're pregnant and you find out late into your pregnancy that the baby you're carrying has

Down syndrome, you're legally entitled to an abortion up until thirty-nine weeks and six days. Yes, really – *thirty-nine weeks and six days*!

I'm not here to tell anyone what to do. I am very open about the fact that I am pro-choice and truly believe everyone has the right to make their own decision. But the message from the top – and by 'the top' I mean the top of the National Health Service and the medical professionals – is that having a baby with DS would be the most awful thing imaginable to happen to you and/ or that in this case, it's totally OK to abort your baby one day before its due date on the grounds that he or she has DS. What is that actually saying?

The use of terminology and language when delivering a diagnosis is so important. Last year a friend of mine sent me a photo of her scan to let me know she was expecting her third child. Underneath the photo she'd noted that she'd asked her midwife to use the word 'chance' rather than 'risk' when referencing her likelihood of having a baby with DS. Now this friend is a good friend. She knows that over the years, like many other parents of children who happen to have Down syndrome, I have gotten a real bee in my bonnet about the use of the word 'risk' and how I'd like it to be replaced. When women go for their first scan around twelve weeks here in the UK, bloods are taken from the expectant mother and a measurement is taken of the fluid behind the baby's neck. From those combined results, that pregnant woman is given her 'risk' of having a baby with Down, Patau or Edwards syndrome: e.g. the risk of you having a baby with Down syndrome may be one in ten thousand, for example. While I understand a lot of women want to screen or indeed go on to have further testing (whether it be the new NIPT or amniocentesis), I've often been puzzled by the use of the word 'risk'. Look up the word 'risk' in the dictionary and you'll see the definition is, 'A situation involving exposure to danger'. Now, the last time I checked, having Oscar hasn't exposed me or anyone else to danger. Quite the opposite, actually. So hence the general feeling that 'chance' would be a much better use of language: 'The chance of you having a baby with Down syndrome is one in ten thousand.'

I was intrigued to know what response my friend received from the midwife when she asked her to use the word 'chance' instead of 'risk'. My friend told me that on the same day she'd seen both a midwife and a sonographer. Apparently, the midwife apologised immediately, exclaiming that she hadn't meant to offend and jotted down in her notes that this was a 'sensitive issue for her'. It wasn't a particularly delicate situation, by the way. My friend, for the record, wasn't too fussed about the screening itself and felt quite bemused that this midwife clearly thought that asking her to use a different term meant she was a tricky patient.

But the sonographer's attitude was quite different. Her response was, 'Yes, but it's a risk assessment. We mean "risk" because it is a risk.' And when my friend exclaimed that it wasn't actually a risk, more that it was a chance, the sonographer's response was that she could still do 'something about it' at twenty weeks, if she'd wanted to.

My friend had been shocked at hearing this. She knew that, legally, she could abort her baby at any point in her pregnancy, if medical practitioners were to find that the child she was carrying did indeed have Down syndrome. But think of the situation in which she was being reminded of this. Here she was, lying on a hospital trolley, being scanned by this healthcare professional. She was taken aback that this is what the advice was, as if aborting the child was no big deal at all.

It could have been the look of outrage on my friend's face or the raised tone of her voice repeating 'still do something *about it*?' that left the sonographer shifting nervously in her seat, stuttering over her words before she just shut up.

I loved my friend's message to me, though, that was the important thing, rather than the responses she received from hospital staff. Who knows if the midwife took on board any of what was said? Perhaps she was more mindful of her language next time – or perhaps she just thought my friend was being oversensitive. I'm not sure the sonographer got it at all, to be honest. It doesn't really sound like it. It sounds like she was too focused on the fact that my friend could 'do something about it' at twenty weeks if she wanted to. Who knows if either of them really *heard* my friend's point. But I shared this exchange on my blog page and the response from it was on another level.

I hoped that there might have been a midwife, sonographer or other healthcare professional out there who read it and had a bit of a lightbulb moment. I hoped they'd see what my friend and I were getting at and that they might change how they approach talking to new mums in the future. The response, however, was more than I could have hoped for. Not only was the blog post shared over and over again, it got thousands of comments and it went viral. I did interviews for both the BBC and ITV News, talking about our personal experience but also about just how important I felt it was that the language healthcare professionals use was not negative or biased. Shortly after – and I'm not crediting my post solely for this, as there were a lot of other people out there making just as much noise – I recieved messages from women who were pregnant, saying that when they'd received paperwork about the screening and testing they could have in the early stages of their pregnancies, they had noticed that the word 'risk' had been replaced by 'chance'. A minor detail to some but a small victory to someone like me, who knew firsthand the impact language can have.

A little while ago I presented a talk to a group of trainee midwives but what I didn't know until afterwards was that a representative from the Royal College of Midwives had been in the lecture theatre listening. He approached me afterwards to say that he found the talk really interesting and that he'd be in touch. I didn't think too much of it until I received an email from his boss who said that he'd spoken to her about the impact of my talk and how, having read more about the work I do, they'd like to add my website and social media channels to the resources page of the 'Delivering unexpected diagnosis' module that every midwife would cover in their training.

When I told my friend I loved her for saying what she did in her appointment and thanked her for at least trying, she wrote back: 'I said those things for you and for Oscar. You are so right and it's such important stuff. You've changed my views on everything (I'm ashamed to say I probably did have the more "typical' mainstream view before you had Ozzie) but now I am so much better educated and see it so differently.'

It's about changing people's mindsets, right? One person at a time. Whether they work in healthcare or whether they're someone like you or I who perhaps didn't have the knowledge and understanding before.

Blog comments

Our daughter had her surgery at five months.
She's eighteen now and we were discharged from
cardiology on Wednesday – for ever. Been a long
time coming, she has never looked back as far as
her heart is concerned.

Anon

I think the best advice – anything and everything
you feel is justified. Allow yourself to worry and
be scared and wonder 'What if?' but remind
yourself you've got this. You've done this. You
know this and there is no one more capable than a
mama who loves her child.

Amy Jayne

CHAPTER FOURTEEN

*'If you think my hands are full,
you should see my heart.'*

I had been worried about 'something going wrong' during both my previous pregnancies and births but when it came to Flo's birth, I can safely say that I did actually manage to relax (well, as much as any pregnant woman can while lying on a table waiting to be sliced open). What I mean, though, was that third time round I finally got the birth I had waited for. The one I had always hoped for. Sure, it wasn't a natural birth, but it was calm and I just had this overwhelming feeling that everything was going to be OK.

Flo slotted into family life fairly easily. I think when you have three children aged three years and under, they kinda sorta have to fit in. She was a fairly chilled baby who would spend a lot of her time watching her troublemaker brothers, who in turn kept her entertained.

Back then I'd often hear the phrase, 'You've got your hands full', when out and about with the three of them. Yep, 'You've got your hands full' – quite possibly the most annoying, overused phrase known to man. Or perhaps it's just me, but you get my gist. I'm talking about the woman in the chemist, the next-door neighbour, the man walking his dog on the street, the midwife, the health visitor, the postman. 'You've got your hands full', always accompanied with a little laugh, like they seriously think they're the first person to come out with this revelation. Sometimes it was delivered with an all-knowing gasp, as in 'You had three children, you nutcase? I stopped at two kids as that was bad enough.' Never one to offend or be rude (I hope), I politely replied with the obligatory chuckle, along with, 'Yes, I know,' when in actual fact what I *really* want to say is, 'No shit, Sherlock!'

The thing is, I *did* indeed have my hands full and just as everyone predicted when I was pregnant, it *was* hard work. And here's the thing. I mean, aside from being pretty knackered from the sleepless nights and experiencing the all-time low of not showering and using a baby wipe to 'freshen up', you know what? I reckon I did all right. I was very much aware that I was never gonna win mother-of-the-year, mind you, but I was doing it. And by 'it' I mean working the mum-of-three thing.

Around the time I had Flo, I did something that I can't say I was proud of. I mean it was a low point in my parenting life so far. I had calculated it and had thought about it before, which probably makes it even worse. I basically lied to make myself look better.

On this day, one of Oscar's therapists was due to visit at 11 a.m. I knew that Alfie would be desperate for his lunch while she was still working with us. He's the type of kid that waits for no one. If he's hungry, he needs feeding, so I needed to be prepared. The last time the therapist had visited, she had asked me about how Alfie's feeding was going and when I said that I used Ella's Kitchen meal pouches, I had felt her judgement at their readymade nature. Knowing she would be turning up when I hadn't made Alfie a 'proper' meal, I decanted one of the Ella's Kitchen packets into a bowl, put clingfilm over it, stashed it in the fridge and when it was time for his lunch I smugly presented it to him (but secretly also her) announcing, 'Here you go, Alfie, here are last night's leftovers for you.'

Mortifying! Yet I'm pleased I did do this, I might add, because as predicted she seemed genuinely interested in what was in said bowl. Thankfully, I got away with it as I explained, 'Oh … it's just pasta, tomatoes (*bugger, what else goes in a meal like this? I scanned the contents of the bowl*) … onion, er, peppers?'

I did this though because I felt guilty. Guilty that I'd

been rubbish and hadn't prepared seven meals for the week on Sunday, frozen them and produced them each mealtime. You may think this sounds ludicrous but there are actual mums out there who bloody well do this. When I told Chris what I'd done, he laughed. He knows me well enough to be aware that my culinary efforts include throwing a supermarket-bought chicken kiev in the oven or chopping an onion for *him* to cook. It got me thinking, though. There are a lot of things in life I feel I'm failing at. Is it an in-built guilt that all mums have? Do we all feel like there's never enough time or, let's face it in this case, inclination, to do the right thing by our children? Throw having a child with additional needs into the equation and I'm wondering if it's heightened even more. I think it just might be.

Rather ridiculously, we moved house when Flo was ten days old. It was, of course, meant to happen months beforehand but, hey, these things never go to plan, right? I had a planned caesarean to get through first. We managed the unpacking *and* the children – with lots of help from family … and copious amounts of wine. Wine helped a lot. Oscar was totally in love with Flo back then and would often go and sit next to her chair and stroke her head or hold her hand. Alfie, on the other hand, was not. He would ignore her most of the time. Every so often, if I'd be feeding her or holding her, he'd go over and give her a little tap or put a bowl/blanket over her head, depending on how the mood took him. I've said it before, but every day was a question of survival. I kinda felt that if we all ended up fed, watered and happy by bedtime then we'd done well. Sometimes, I felt that having three kids, one of them was always missing out. Like, if I spent too much time playing with the boys, Flo would end up being neglected but then equally, if my attention turned to Flo for too long, Oscar and Alfie would more than likely end up getting up to mischief together.

I think that's one of people's biggest fears when they have a child with a disability. That the other sibling (or others) are going to miss out, be neglected or ignored. And while I'm not gonna lie, on occasion, like the time Chris took all three to the skate park to give them a whiz around on their scooters and lost Flo (by then aged three) for some five minutes because he was too busy chasing after Oscar, who was then heading at speed into the nearby children's playground. But I can hand on heart say that the positives of having Oscar in Alfie and Flo's lives outweigh the losing-them-in-skate-park-type situations.

I recall when I first had Flo, wondering if my house would ever be tidy again. Would I ever make a meal from scratch (not that I ever did but I might one day, right?)? Would I ever sit down in the evenings and relax again? Around 5 p.m. Flo would decide she didn't want to be put down and needed to be fussed over or fed constantly (a hard time of the day, when I also needed to get two boys their tea and get them ready for bed). Around this time all hell was always in danger of breaking loose and after 7 p.m., the boys' bedtime, I would normally need my me-time or want to talk to Chris. Now, I had Flo, still fussing and feeding until she'd finally give in and go to sleep.

That was another thing I learnt about having Oscar and then having the other two. Oscar lulled me into this false sense of security as he was literally the dream baby. He never used to really cry, went down to bed in the evenings and slept all night from around the age of eight weeks. I even remember my health visitor insisting I woke him for feeds because he was a low birth-weight and at the time not gaining that fast. She was adamant that's what I should do. I think I maybe tried it for a couple of nights but he was so dozy and didn't want to feed then, plus all the other mums I knew were saying, 'Are you mad! Why would you wake him if he doesn't wake – take the goddamn sleep while you can.'

I do think I came to the realisation around the time I had Flo that, when he wasn't sleeping, Oscar literally never stopped. And maybe it was also because I was trying to juggle looking after a newborn and two toddlers, but Oscar, as lovely as he was, required a different level of care. And I know a lot of people are going to say, 'He was three, Sarah. That's normal three-year-old behaviour,' and to a point they'd be right. Yet the difference became really obvious when I compared the times that I'd have just Alfie and Flo because Oz would be in nursery with the days I had Oscar and Flo while Alfie was at his nursery. When Oscar was around, I saw that I couldn't ever really let my guard down.

That's not to say that Alfie was easy. He wasn't. He understood exactly what was asked of him. He tantrum-ed with the best of them and, if left to his own devices, would have run off at the drop of a hat. He was saying a few words at this point but equally got frustrated that I wouldn't understand what he'd be trying to tell me. He acted, I suspect, just as any other twenty-one-month child might do but I think the difference was that I could read Alfie a little better. Whereas Oscar, well, he was just that little more unpredictable.

Although Oscar would understand what was asked of him, sometimes he'd get sidetracked. I could ask him to go and get his shoes but if there'd be something interesting on the way to picking up his shoes, that would have taken his attention and the shoes would be forgotten. His energy levels were always high and, at times, managing that energy was tough. And that's not to say he wasn't doing well but I realised there were a lot of things he still did at this point that other three-year-olds had grown out of. For example, if I wasn't looking, he'd sit and take out all the baby wipes from a packet, just because he could. Or if we'd been in the park, I'd have to shadow him the whole time, just in case he'd run out of the gate and dart across the road. And if for a moment I took my eyes off him, even for a couple of seconds, he could just decide to lie down in the park and lick the tarmac, which, honestly, is just gross and so uncalled for, don't you think?

What I'm trying to say is that, yes, Alfie was a handful at his age but, if all went as it 'typically' should, I knew he would grow out of it. We knew we wouldn't always have to watch him as closely as we did and, in time, we could relax. Yes, Flo was a newborn and relied on me for everything, but again this I knew would be over in the blink of an eye. Which left me wondering – would Oscar always need to be watched so closely?

I spoke recently to another mum of a little girl who happened to have DS. Her daughter was thirteen and has one older and one younger sister. They had visited Florida and had been to Disney's Typhoon Lagoon water park and the mum commented that this was the first time she'd trusted her thirteen-year-old to stay with her sisters if they went off together. It was also the first time she'd been conscious of her daughter asking to go to the bathroom alone and letting her go. As I write this, Oscar has just turned six and that still seems so far off for us. But as I said, his time will come

– we're just still so unsure of how long that time will take to arrive.

Our house is relatively Oscar-proof these days and for the most part he's so much more sensible than he used to be, but there are still times now when I will leave him downstairs and still listen out for what he's up to. In the last year he's gone into one of my kitchen cupboards, got the sugar and just decided to pour the entire contents onto the floor. Why? I have no bloody idea – but it was another gentle reminder not to ever let my guard down.

Anyway, I know all parents worry about their children's welfare and this isn't meant to come across as me being all doom-and-gloom but I guess it's about looking at the facts. At that time I had three very young children. One had additional needs and needed me to be his protector. It wasn't about wishing the time away, because believe me, every evening I sat with Flo having her fussy five minutes (hours), I'd look into that little face of hers and soak up every second because I knew she wouldn't be that teeny baby in my arms for long (and because, seriously, there was absolutely no chance in hell I was having any more kids). And when Alfie had a meltdown because he'd been expecting to watch *Peter Rabbit* and not the episode of *Postman Pat* I'd put on for him, I'd try really hard to keep calm and remember it wouldn't be too long before he could tell me *exactly* what he wanted.

But when it came to Oz, no matter how brilliantly he was doing, I realised time was going to move a little more slowly for the two of us. I'd wanted him to stay small so I would always be there to protect him and not have to think too much about the future or what lay ahead for him but sometimes, if I'm truly honest, I wished it was just that little bit easier. Not just for me, but for him.

I always knew having three would be hard and although Oscar and Alfie were pretty equal at that point in the amount of care they'd needed, albeit in slightly different ways, I guess I knew that with Alfie it'd probably pass a lot quicker than with Oz. And it did.

I wouldn't know for some time what the future held for him (and here I am now, still wondering) but it was about trying to live in the moment rather than worrying about too far ahead. Yes, at times I felt run ragged and, yes, at times the guilt I felt was all-consuming – about thinking I should do more or spend more quality time with all my children – but seeing them all together and all happy was worth every second I spent picking Oscar up from the tarmac.

So what I'm saying is, life can be hard sometimes but this *is* my life and when I look around, comparing my existence to what some people go through, it isn't all bad.

Blog comments

I love your page and all the things you and your beautiful children get up to. I thought of you today; I mentioned to a friend that my son had recently had an ADHD diagnosis, and she said, 'Oh, I'm really sorry to hear that.'

The words that left my mouth were, 'Don't be sorry, it's not that awful!'

Since having my son and realising he has ADHD, and having a diagnosis, I've realised that there is a massive lack of understanding in the world with regard to any form of SEN. People need to understand they all have so much potential and they are all gifted in more ways than many people without SEN are. I work in early years anyway, so I'm used to seeing children from all walks of life. I hope one day it's all less of a taboo.

Sian Walker

Hi, Sarah. I've been reading your blog for maybe a year now. I love the way you write totally from the heart. Your kids are all just beautiful and I love seeing the pictures you take of them. Earlier this year, in April, at thirteen weeks' pregnant we received a devastating prognosis for our baby.

He/she had extensive fluid around the head, neck and shoulder area, a cystic hygroma. We were told our baby had a very low chance of survival and probably had a 'genetic condition'. Being the types who seek answers before making any decisions, John – my husband – and I decided to go for further tests to understand what we were dealing with (NIPT and amnio). Bear in mind we live in Ireland where abortion was illegal and we were also in the midst of a controversial abortion referendum [the ban on abortion was overturned by 66.4 per cent of the votes cast in May 2018]. Not the nicest of times. You can imagine the posters! Results of amnio confirmed the NIPT 'risk' (chance) that our baby had T21/DS. I have always been very pro-choice on these matters but I (we) were faced with a decision.

I have had a lot of experience of teens and young adults with DS as my mum worked as a teacher for children and teens with additional needs, primarily DS. My husband, through contact with our family, has also had some exposure. However, I did worry if our family could cope with this despite all the support. We made the decision, very easily, to keep the baby and I'm now twenty-eight weeks pregnant. We also have two little girls, Grace (seven) and Sarah (four) who now know a baby is coming but know nothing of the diagnosis. The baby (we don't know the sex) also has a complete AVSD (similar to Oscar?) and will require surgery at three/four months which I'm nervous about but the medics are very reassuring. Bizarrely, also, the fluid has disappeared and pregnancy is relatively normal at this stage! We are coping well and managing the diagnosis within our own little family, plus my own family who also know. We have only told some good friends so far.

I suppose the reason I'm messaging you is because of that story you posted the other day about the lady who had wished she found your blog sooner. You assumed that she had possibly had a termination. The story really struck me and I sent it on to John who replied with 'We have totally made the right decision'. To be honest, I'm not sure we really made a 'decision' as when we discovered our baby had DS we both agreed very quickly that we were going to continue the pregnancy, without much discussion. I know that you never had that decision with Oscar's postnatal diagnosis. I know I'm rambling here but I wanted to let you know that despite the fact that I had found your blog before we faced our own journey, it has put many smiles on my face over the last few months. You seem to be a very normal mum with the same struggles and ups and downs we all experience. You're doing an amazing job of educating people and I imagine it does influence people's decision-making. So well done and keep up the good work and keep taking those gorgeous pictures of your monkeys!

Sinéad O'Brien

CHAPTER FIFTEEN

'A mother's love for her child is like nothing else in the world. It knows no law, no pity, it dares all things and crushes down remorselessly all that stands in its path.'

– AGATHA CHRISTIE, 'THE LAST SÉANCE',
THE HOUND OF DEATH AND OTHER STORIES, 1933

In October 2015, I received a letter in the post. A letter that quite honestly left me feeling sick to my stomach. The local authority told me that Oscar was to be denied an EHCP (Education Health and Care Plan) assessment that we needed in place before he started school.

He had been due to start school in September 2016 and the EHCP process was the new name for the 'statement' that used to be issued to a child. We had applied on the advice of some of the professionals who worked with Oscar to ensure that he had one-to-one education from a teaching assistant when he began. The

EHCP gathers evidence from those closely involved in the child's life, including therapists, professionals and parents or carers to try to prove that the extra support is necessary. What the letter meant, in short, was that Oscar's needs were currently being met at his nursery. We had the FEET funding in place and extra funding for a few hours of one-to-one at the nursery and so they had ruled that further assessment was not required.

Like most parents of a little one approaching school age, we had started to think where we'd like Oscar to go. For some children it might be quite straightforward – are they in the right catchment area? Has the school got a good Ofsted (Office for Standards in Education) rating? I think that in most cases the question of where to place your child is not one that parents take lightly, but when you add in to the mix that we have a child with Down syndrome or for those with any other additional needs, it can raise a whole heap of questions and concerns – oh, and a ridiculous amount of form-filling and paperwork!

Parents of a child with DS have to decide from the outset about whether to send their child to mainstream school or a special school. I found it interesting in speaking to a number of friends and acquaintances when we were thinking about it. Most of them would ask, with caution and trepidation, what we were planning to do with Oscar. I obviously didn't mind the question. It was a completely valid one, after all. But I did wonder why they asked it with such care. I guess no one liked to automatically assume he'd be going to mainstream school. Perhaps people asked the question with the same mindset I had back when I went to school – believing that there just weren't people with DS in mainstream education, or very few at least. If that was the case, perhaps those people would be surprised (and I hope pleased) to hear that between 80 and 90 per cent of children with DS start out in a mainstream school these days.

For our kids, as you know, it's all about early intervention and the fact that there is proof that with the right support, children with DS are learning to read and write just as their peers do, even if it does take that little bit longer. There is a lot of evidence to suggest that putting kids like Oscar in their own age group helps to aid their development. It was always my hope that in doing so everyone involved would also gain a greater understanding of DS and other learning difficulties and any preconceived misconceptions would be wiped out … eventually. I know this is still a work-in-progress but I hope it will happen, even if it does take a few more years to filter through.

We know that our kids respond better to a visual learning style. We also know that visual processing and visual memory skills are a strength of children with DS. That's why there's proof that reading is usually a relative strength. We know that social understanding is something that our children are good at and that non-verbal communication, such as Makaton, is an area they excel in. We know that they are more than likely going to have specific speech and language delays. Their receptive language is usually superior to expressive language (in other words, their ability to understand words and language is usually better than their speaking) and their auditory short-term memory and auditory processing are areas of weakness. Auditory short-term memory is the ability to take in information orally and retain it. Auditory processing is what the brain does to make sense of sound.

If a mainstream school was aware of all the points above relating to Oscar and a teaching assistant was good at his or her job (in our case, working alongside his therapists and me in setting him targets to achieve greater things), then the process of inclusion I believed would absolutely work. I had all this in the back of my mind when Chris and I first started thinking about Oscar's education and what would be right for him. It was our hope that he would attend a mainstream school and, perhaps naively at first, in my quest to find the right setting I thought inclusion and integration would be the ethos of every mainstream school. I had been mistaken.

Our local primary school, which we'd always hoped Oscar would attend, was our first choice. There were other schools in the area that we'd liked, too, and we were so pleased we had options to consider. However, there was one school in particular, also close to us, which advertised 'inclusion' but, honestly, couldn't have made it any clearer that *their* 'inclusion' didn't extend to *our* son – they didn't want Oscar there. I guess as parents, you have a few filed questions that you bring out when testing whether a setting is the right place for your child.

When we met them, I said that with Oscar being a summer-born baby (July), he would have only just turned four when he started school and while I would do my upmost to have him dry (toilet trained) the likelihood was that he would still be in pull-ups. My question was about the provisions the school would make, should that be the case. I'd hoped the person we spoke to would say that it wouldn't be a problem and that they'd have facilities to change him. But the response of this lady – who, by the way, was the assistant head teacher and SENCo– was to remind me that 'with him being a summer-born baby, you know you can defer his entry'.

Of course I knew this but it angered me that she hadn't answered my question. I had asked what provision they'd make for his toileting, not given her an excuse to say why he shouldn't attend. The rest of the meeting I recall went along the same lines.

I had walked around the school and seen a little boy with ear defenders on (who the teacher pointed out had autism). He had his back to the class, his head in his hands and was sat quietly on his own. She had said he got quite overwhelmed at times and that was why he was there. If this was their idea of inclusion then in that instant I knew this wouldn't be the place for my son. In response to everything I asked that day, I got a sense that Oscar would have been a burden for them. I left feeling sad but mainly very cross that they had publicised their spiel about integration and inclusion, but the reality was they blatantly didn't want Oscar. In hindsight I'm only glad they were so very obvious about it because it made our decision about where *not* to send him a very easy one.

They talk about a gut feeling you get when it comes to choosing a setting for your child and I'm a firm believer in that. We looked around specialist provisions just to get a comparison but we believed mainstream was in Oscar's best interests at that time. We also always agreed that if at any point we felt that he was struggling or unhappy, then we would of course reassess.

As for the letter I received that morning about the assessment? I tried all day to get hold of the lady who wrote it. I wanted to let her know that just because Oscar's needs were being met in nursery at the moment, it didn't mean he shouldn't be assessed for the way in which his needs would be met at school. I wanted to let her know that I wouldn't just sit back and accept this because Oscar (and others like him) have the right to at least try in mainstream education.

A lot of children with additional needs who started school in the year before Oscar did so without an EHCP in place. The process was in its first year and there were definitely teething problems. Many schools had to appoint TAs (teaching assistants), at a cost they had to bear themselves, because having accepted a child with DS into the school they felt it was their duty of care to make sure that the child was well looked-after. As I said, we had been told by various professionals to submit our form in September 2015, when he was three (which we did) only to be advised by the authority who received it that it was too soon. I worried that, like many school-starters that year, in leaving it too much longer we would miss out because the submission would be too late.

We had been told that Oscar, and children like him, could have anything from thirteen to thirty-three hours of support a week. It was very varied and obviously depended on each individual child's needs. It had been our hope that Oscar would have the complete thirty-three hours of full-time one-to-one support (or as close to it as possible). Thirteen hours (the minimum that councils have been known to allocate), in my opinion, just wouldn't be sufficient. I wouldn't have let it happen.

Oscar had started his visits to the preschool room at nursery that same week we received the letter. By all accounts, it was going well, but his key worker said to me one morning that he was very excitable and into everything. It was very hard to separate what exactly was just Oscar – a three-year-old boy exploring his new surroundings – and what was the DS. I was told that the snack table was now on show the whole time and readily available to him. He would play, then go over for a snack and had a tendency to play with the knives on the table.

Now we were faced with making a final decision about where to send him, a whole heap of questions were flying around my head – would he cope in mainstream school? It was hard to imagine Oscar ever 'calming down' and not being quite so excitable, but then I had to remind myself that some of my friends felt exactly the same way about their children with DS when they entered a mainstream school, and they seemingly were doing well. The thought of Oscar conforming and doing what he was told was daunting. Should I think about keeping him back a year, seeing as he was a summer-born baby? Perhaps with an extra year in preschool and him then being one of the oldest in the year, would mean that the gap in development wouldn't be quite so wide? Should I send him to a special school instead? But then he'd miss out entirely on mainstream. Would I be doing him a disservice by not trying or would I be making a mistake by sending him to mainstream education only to find that he didn't manage?

I didn't believe there actually was a generic right or wrong answer as far as special or mainstream was concerned. All I could do is select the school that was right for my child, he was an individual, after all. That was all any parent could do. Every one of us has a right to an education and as long as Oscar was happy, I'd be happy. That was surely all there was to it.

It was with the right support in place that Oscar would thrive. He'd be allowed to learn, explore, watch others, socialise and integrate just as any other little person does when they start school. I just hoped that the EHCP process would be finalised as quickly and as painlessly as possible. I had no idea at this point just how many hoops I'd have to jump through to get there. I'd been thankful for the parents who'd been there and done it and were sharing information to help people like me. I thanked my friends who were currently going through the same thing and who had given me a kick up the butt to get things moving. Without them, all this would have been a lot more daunting.

I was told that our local authority made it harder for us because there were always going to be parents who sat back and accepted what they're given, even if it wasn't enough for their child. The authorities are relying on the fact that some people will do just that, even if the one-to-one sessions are too few to give their child the attention they need. I have always worried about those children. Not because they're not loved but because their parents haven't necessarily got the fight in them. They haven't perhaps got the skills to collate the reports they need, the know-how in filling out all the relevant forms. I have always worried, and still do, about what happens to those kids? And it breaks my heart.

I knew back then that I wasn't going to be one of those parents. I simply couldn't be or else I truly believe I would have failed my little boy.

Blog comments

Hi. I was told about your page by a friend of a friend who is a special-needs nanny. I'd been put in touch with her as we have just had a little girl, Ruby, with Down's. I was 'high risk' in pregnancy with a one-in-four chance but didn't do any further testing to get the definitive answer. Mainly because I didn't want to risk a miscarriage and because it wouldn't have stopped me continuing. Ruby was postnatally diagnosed and actually Lewisham, London, hospital staff never used any negative language with us. Lucky. Maybe they've changed. Ruby is one month old now and we are slowly learning about what it all might mean for us. We have another daughter who is seventeen months and doesn't have Down's. I've just read lots of your posts – pretty much all of my emotions and thoughts are in there somewhere! It's been a bit overwhelming so far with health things and if I'm honest I've not arrived at any place yet acceptance-wise or joy-wise, if that makes sense? I really want to get to a place where I don't wish that she was healthy/normal/typical – what are the right words? I hope that doesn't offend you. Thanks for your posts, I'll keep reading. And I am looking forward to us all getting to know Ruby and not just worrying about her health and future, etc. Sorry for such a brain dump but wanted to say thanks for being so honest – it really helps!

Jeni Noel

Hi, Sarah. I am writing to you tonight because I am feeling … so many things. Angry, sad, helpless and … mute. Like I don't have a voice to fight for my child. In the early days of having our daughter, Isobel, at home, I read your blog and it gave immense comfort to me. I wrote to you about how your blog had really helped me. I guess that's why I am turning to you again tonight. Today our nursery of choice for Isobel told us she cannot go there. There is an issue with funding for her and they will not accept her any more. I go back to work a week tomorrow. This is a bombshell. I feel as if the rug has been pulled from beneath us and I feel so angry at the injustice of how they can turn their back on my little beauty. I have asked the nursery to review the decision. We have offered to pay the shortfall in funding should it be awarded (essentially there is a discrepancy between funding for those under one and over).

I have sat with Isobel during three settling-in sessions last week and watched how she has responded to the new environment positively. Then I left her by herself for her fourth session and on my return she was sat at the snack table while the other children ate. She wasn't eating, she is exclusively fed with an NG (nastrogastric) tube. Her key person said, 'I know she can't eat with them but I wanted her to sit with her friends.' I felt this was wonderful – the key person got it. She understood the importance of including Isobel. We had community nursing on site to sign off the key person to feed Isobel and it was all going well. But now, that feeling of comfort, of thinking Isobel had a chance of being positively involved in this setting, has gone. She has been singled out as a burden. I am beside myself because I want so much for her to thrive in this environment. I don't know what I want from you but I suppose when you are at a low point you return to the place that gave you comfort. So we await the nursery's final decision. They have said that Isobel can go as planned for a month in order to allow us to make alternative arrangements. So tomorrow I will drop her off for her first day. It was supposed to be a day of excitement for her and me – instead it feels rubbish.

Sarah Mayes

CHAPTER SIXTEEN

'The greatest wealth is health.'

– VIRGIL

There's a big old debate that often gets bashed out within the DS community about whether or not, if they could, parents would take the DS away if they could.

Some say, 'My child is who they are because of the DS.' Others say, 'My child isn't defined by who they are because they happen to have the condition.' There is a part of me that thinks that Oscar is so much more than the label and diagnosis. But then the DS does make him different. It does mean he finds things harder than others. So if I had the chance, would I take it away?

What I am one hundred per cent certain about, and I can say with more certainty than before, is that I would absolutely take away the health-related issues Oscar has that are associated with being a person who happens to have DS. And I know some will say that any child could be born with a hole in the heart and any child could get glue ear, any boy could have an undescended testicle and any child can have an underactive thyroid (all of which Oscar has) but there's of course more likelihood that a person who has DS is going to have these things,

Oscar has always suffered with ear problems. As I touched on earlier, he had had the BAHA (bone-anchored hearing aid) for a short time and all the while he actually wore it, it really helped his hearing. The older he got, though, the more I felt it became a hinderance more than a help. Oscar got wise to the fact that it was a brilliant distraction technique in therapy sessions: *If I toss this across the room, the speech therapist is going to stop what she's doing to retrieve it, resulting in a little break for me.* As I said, he's not stupid, this kid. So having heard success stories from other parents who had little ones with DS, we decided that grommets might be a better option for helping to clear his glue ear and aid his hearing. Around the same time that Flo was born we asked to be referred to an ENT (ear, nose and throat) consultant to talk about the possibility. Oscar had had an audiology appointment to check his hearing again. They'd found in some areas his hearing had gotten better, but in others a little worse. They said the loss was moderate (as it seemingly had always been) and that the key thing was that he was still congested, due to having the glue ear.

So I had this meeting with the ENT consultant where I'd hoped he'd make the decision for us. The thing I've learnt over the years, though, is that as Oscar's parents, we ultimately have the final say. Unless something is life and death, it's our choice what we do. A doctor cannot sway us either way. This one told me the pros and cons of grommets. He said he could absolutely do the procedure but that there were no guarantees and that there would be risks involved (they could fall out or cause damage to the ear drum). If they worked, however, Oscar's hearing and development could drastically improve so, really, I left no clearer about what the right thing would be to do for him.

I recall Chris and I deciding between us that perhaps we would leave it a few more months and really persevere with making him wear his BAHA; *if* he managed to keep the band on, he'd hear so much better and this would obviously help with his speech. Feeling determined, as we left the hospital I purposefully put the band on him and hoped for the best. Needless to say, between the audiology department and the car park he probably took it off about ten times and either handed it to me or tried to give it to random passersby but we gave it a good go.

We persisted with the hated BAHA band and there

seemed to be a shift and it actually worked for a while. Either it was because he was just that bit older or it was because he'd finally realised that in keeping it on he could hear better. For a while we noticed a change in his concentration levels. He used more Makaton signs and was even attempting more words. We carried on for about six months but still had to spend time going and back forth to the hospital because he did still keep taking the band off, throwing it away and breaking the damn thing. I was exasperated and decided that maybe grommets actually were the best option. We got another ENT appointment. Thinking I was probably going to have a fight on my hands, as the consultant had been reluctant to book him in for the op last time, on meeting for the second time, I started by explaining we had been having terrible trouble with Oscar keeping the band on. As if on cue, Oscar threw it across the room (seriously, it couldn't have been timed better). I thought the consultant might still be reluctant but he actually said we could give grommets a go!

We were well aware that grommets don't always work and that there was always the risk that the ear drum could be perforated, but the positives, for us, outweighed the negatives at this point. For me, it was about giving Oscar the opportunity to hear better. If they fell out and he needed to wear the aid later down the line then so be it – at least we would have given it a go!

We only had to wait a month before he was called in for the surgery, although unfortunately, all didn't go completely to plan. The team managed to insert one of the grommets into the right ear, but when they went to do the left ear, they found a large cluster of skin cells called cholesteatoma and that took us on a completely different path as far as his ears were concerned. The plan was to do a CT scan with Oscar under sedation to allow them to take a look at the extent of the growth, working out where it was and what had been affected in the ear canal, ear drum and hearing-wise, etc. Then we were told he'd need another surgery under general anaesthetic to remove the growth and then, potentially, more surgery to sort out the hearing at a later date. They couldn't tell at this point if the hearing had been affected in that ear but would know more after they'd taken out the growth. They were confident though, that they had caught it early. He was still only three and wasn't showing any symptoms of leaky ears, dizziness or facial paralysis – which was obviously a good sign. If left untreated, we were told, the cholesteatoma could cause damage to the ear canal. This might mean his hearing could get worse so, basically, they needed to get it out.

The surgeon said the condition wasn't something that was necessarily associated with having DS but it was more complicated because of their smaller ear canals. In the days that followed, I obviously did more research.

I googled, joined forums and read up about it. I think at the time the ENT surgeon had told me the news it had been too much to take in and it wasn't until further investigation that I realised how big a deal this could potentially be. It felt like yet another hurdle my little man would have to face. I mean I know he'd smashed life so far but seriously, give him a break.

We decided there would be no harm in letting him settle into school before the procedure, so he actually didn't end up having it done until January 2017. It took five hours and thirty minutes – longer than first anticipated and a lengthier op that even his open-heart surgery had been when he was a little baby. To me, this latest surgery literally felt like it took *for ever*. I don't think I've ever drunk so much coffee in my life as we sat waiting in the hospital cafe. I wouldn't even go out into the grounds of the hospital much less leave the premises for fear of something going wrong and not being there. Chris had wanted to sit outside on the warm day in January, so I watched him from the window of the cafe, worried that the pager wouldn't work if I joined him.

Thankfully, all went well. They managed to get the cholesteatoma out and were happy with the results but they did acknowledge that it'd been very difficult. Oscar's ears were so tiny and it was intricate work. They told us there was a chance that it could grow back, which meant that he'd need follow-up surgery in nine months to see how it was going. Oscar also had packing in his ear for three weeks and we were told he'd only be able to hear out of the other ear and would need to come back to have the packing removed (again, under general anaesthetic).

One piece of very good news was that the surgeon had managed to insert a titanium implant, as the disease had eroded a lot of the components that make up the ear, meaning that in time Oscar could get his hearing back. So, yes, as I said, that was the start of Oscar's Ear Journey. It's been a long one and I could probably write another book on what has happened since but I'll leave it for now and update you in book no. 2!

This leads me back to Oscar's heart. You guys thought that was all fixed, right? Well, it was. It is. Except that, in the course of having regular heart check-ups every six to nine months after the surgery – slowly increasing to every nine months, then yearly – we were hit with the bombshell that his lungs were now under strain and he had something called pulmonary hypertension. This was increased blood pressure in the lungs. In October 2014, when Oscar was just two years old, he was referred to the respiratory clinic at the Royal Brompton Hospital, London. He'd had a sleep study done a few weeks prior and it flagged up that he had very mild sleep apnoea, pauses or gaps in breathing overnight. They said they felt that the apnoea wasn't the reason that Oscar's lungs were under strain but they were now wondering what was the root cause. They explored the chest, which looked clear, and suggested that he be referred to ENT (again) so that they could take a look at his tonsils to see if they were enlarged, causing an obstruction and therefore affecting the lungs. The other option was referring him to their SALT to assess his swallow (for reflux/silent aspiration).

So we did follow up with all these appointments. It turned out that the cause of the lung problem was indeed the swallow rather than the apnoea, chest or his tonsils. Oscar had a videofluoroscopy, again at the Brompton, where he had to sit in a chair and drink from his cup (while watching *Mister T* on their DVD player, which, thankfully, distracted him). In the cup, they'd put a special liquid that the radiographer, team of speech therapists and doctor could track on the X-ray. You'd imagine it would take a while to see if the liquid was going down where it was meant to, but it needed only one sip for them to see that Oscar had silent aspiration – meaning that while the majority of the drink went down the correct way, a little seeped into his windpipe. This basically explained the strain on his lungs (pulmonary hypertension) and accounted for the fact that he'd been susceptible to chest infections over the previous few years.

The SALT said I might have noticed that when Oscar took a sip of a drink, he would sometimes look wide-

and watery-eyed. He had a little if I thought about it but I certainly didn't remember noticing it too much. They'd been no coughing or spluttering – but I guess that was why they called it silent aspiration. Oscar was prescribed a thickening powder which was to be added to every drink from then on. It was their hope that by changing the consistency, it'd take more time, the liquid being that much thicker, for him to swallow it, thus allowing him to control where the liquid went. It all made sense. People with DS have low muscle tone, as I've mentioned before, and so it was fairly common for little ones to have this problem. The muscles in their throat are so relaxed that it's no wonder this occurs sometimes. I was relieved to have gotten an answer as to why his lungs could have been under strain and we were told if we persisted with the thickener, over time the lungs should sort themselves out.

So – yeah, over the years there have been some shit times, if I'm honest. I mean, obviously I'm thankful that we've not had anything too major but there have been a number of times I've thought, this is all a bit rubbish. To go back to the question I asked at the beginning of the chapter – would I change the DS? It's not really about changing the DS. The DS I can actually cope with. It's all the associated issues that go with the diagnosis that are stressful. The growth in his ear was just rotten luck but I guess the silent aspiration was a result of having

DS. All I have ever wanted for Oscar is for life to be a bit easier. For him to not have to face the hurdles he's had to. But do you know what? Every time he's had any new health-related problem, he always goes into it with strength and determination and regularly smashes it out the park.

Blog comments

I pray to god I learn to accept that this was our fate. I pray that I fall in love with my son eventually. I pray that I learn to love our life again and take pleasure in the littlest things and I pray to god he has a happy and healthy life and is an independent little person. It's been seven weeks. When will I ever accept it?

Harps Kaur

Hi, I don't know why I am messaging you, perhaps because you seem like such a positive person. I found out two weeks ago that I'm expecting a baby with Down syndrome. Since the diagnosis I feel a sense of overwhelming sadness that I cannot seem to shake off.

Ciara Flynn

CHAPTER SEVENTEEN

'Expectation feeds frustration.'
– STEVE MARABOLI

In the January before Oscar started school, we were walking past our local park when Oscar started pointing and shouting about the fact that he'd like to go in and play. I didn't really think about the fact that it also happened to be around the same time as the local primary school had finished for the day and we went in.

Clearly delighted that his wish had come true, he proceeded to run around, asking me for help (albeit in his own way) when he couldn't quite manage something. He was loving it and super-excited. Perhaps a little over-excited and I'm going to say something now that's probably a little controversial and isn't going to sit well with some, but he was doing his 'excitable Down syndrome thing'. Now, I do not want to say that all kids with DS do this, but it's just something that Oscar has always done. When he's excited, he breathes in and out of his nose *really* fast. As I said, he's always done it, from a very young age, but now he was three and a half and other kids of that age don't act this way. It was really obvious that this is his 'DS thing'.

All of a sudden, I felt people were looking at him. To be honest with you, I don't think I'd felt this for a long time, but I felt their stares that day. Groups of women were looking over. Some were smiling, some were doing that sideways look, where it was as if they were pretending not to but they obviously were while trying not to seem rude, and then some were just blatantly staring. Perhaps they were intrigued, perhaps they'd never seen a child with DS in the park before, but all of a sudden I felt very alone. I'd considered myself a fairly confident person. I think probably more so since having Oscar so, normally, I'd be one to hold my head high but that day, it seemed I couldn't. Instead, after a few minutes (and because it was also bloody freezing) we left. To add insult to injury, Oscar, who didn't want to leave, went into meltdown and wouldn't go in the pushchair. He was rigid and defiant and all I was thinking was that I bet those women were now stood there feeling bad for me. Thinking something along the lines of, Aah, look at her with her special needs son … how sad. And I hated that I was thinking that.

I felt annoyed. Not with them really. I got that people were going to be curious, but I felt annoyed that this was probably how the next however many years were going to go. Was I really going to have to explain my son to others and explain why he did the things he did? I was cross with myself that evening. Not just because I fled the park but because I realised I'd left because I'd felt embarrassed. I guess some days, regardless of how strong a person you normally feel you are, sometimes there's no fight left in you. I think that day I was tired (I was probably on a diet knowing me, so we'll blame the lack of sugar) but I was annoyed that I'd let others get to me.

There was no doubt that Oscar's communication was really coming on. We'd heard a few more words recently and his signing seemed to be evolving all the time, but as far as speech was concerned, he was definitely an 'I'll do it in my own time' kind of a kid. It didn't worry me back then, I don't think. I'd heard from others that some kiddies with DS had little or no speech at this stage and then once they started school, they took off. But I know that on occasions such as when we were in the park, I felt sad from time to time when his frustrations came into play.

We'd have Oscar's friends to our house sometimes. They were all 'typical' kids and had known Oscar for a while and I'd watch as they all played. Some played in pairs. Some played alone. But I'd watch and see that although Oscar tried desperately to join in, he often got left behind. I remember one of the boys once even gave Oscar a toy to play with. It was a kind gesture so I said to Oscar, 'Say "thank you".' I always say 'say' (even now) but for the most part he couldn't actually 'say' what I was asking him to. More often than not, he'd sign what I was asking and in this case he did just that. But the little boy he was talking to turned to me, looked me straight in the eye and said, 'Oscar can't say "thank you" because he can't talk yet'. And he'd been right. He couldn't say 'thank you'. Which I guess in contrast to his other friends, it would appear that he couldn't say much at all. But that kid that day floored me. I mean, it was like a punch to the stomach. The cold, hard truth delivered by a three-and-a-half-year-old. Don't get me wrong, he'd been absolutely right in what he'd been saying but my god did it hurt.

I'm guessing his mummy, my lovely friend, had spoken to him about the fact that Oscar couldn't say much yet. I'm guessing she did indeed 'teach' him just that. I found myself that day reiterating what she had probably already told him, that Oscar would talk one day, we hope, and that it'll just take him a little longer and there I was again, just as I'd expected I'd have to, teaching the world (in this case a three-and-a-half-year-old) about my child.

I promised myself not to do the whole comparison thing. I don't know how many times I'd sit talking to Chris or to my mum, telling them that I wasn't going to compare Oscar to typical kids his age but how could I not, back then? I think it felt heightened as since Alfie had turned two, his speech had suddenly come on. I mean obviously I'd never had a 'typically developing' child before (and, believe me, I'm not saying Alfie was the next Einstein) but my god, I remember thinking how the hell did he know all those words? I had sat with Oscar through endless therapy sessions, practising our words and matching our pictures. For hours! And then Alfie would swoop in and just says things, just like that. Things that I hadn't even taught him to say. Like 'moon'. For some reason that sticks in my mind. We'd gotten out the car after nursery one night, he'd pointed to the sky and shouted, '*Moooon, mummy.*' How?

What I know is that I have never come across another parent of a child with Down syndrome who leads anything other than a normal, happy life. Sure, there are challenges but then there are in life regardless, right? And I guess I do repeatedly teach the world about my child. I feel like I owe it to him to show others just how great a life he leads. Had we had a prenatal diagnosis, at that point I wouldn't have been able to see how our lives would be – fear of the unknown would have got in the way.

I guess I was still teaching him about the world, too. Albeit slowly. He'd get there eventually, I knew that. But more importantly than teaching the world about my child, he was teaching me things every single day.

Blog comments

I'm nineteen weeks pregnant today and last Thursday, after having the SAFE (non-invasive prenatal) test, we found out that we have a 95 per cent chance of having a baby with Down syndrome. Tomorrow we go back to speak to the specialist midwife about the results and the future. It's been so good to see your family as our hearts are desperate to welcome our baby into the world. No need to reply, just wanted to say thank you.

Polly Hannah

Hello, Sarah, I've been plucking up the courage to message you for weeks, so please don't think it's something I do lightly. I've spent many hours reading your page and blogs, and your strength and energy as a mother astounds me. Your overarching passion is to raise a greater awareness of DS and you show resilience daily in dealing with people who are not as knowledgeable or are misinformed on what it means to have DS or raise a child that happens to have it. I'm afraid I was one of those ill-informed people. My world fell apart in December when, having told everyone I was pregnant (with our second) I got a call to say my bloods and NT had come back as 'high risk' and that I had a one-in-thirty chance of giving birth to a baby with DS. We had the amnio test. And the day before Christmas (5.38 p.m.) we got a call to say it was a definite. We were naturally shocked and felt very alone. It might pain (even disgust) you to hear that I went on to have a termination.

Sarah, I'm not looking for your forgiveness, or anything of that nature. Why am I even writing to you, you wonder? It's because you clearly have a voice and a passion to raise an awareness of DS. And if there was something I'd like to come of this horrid situation that I'll carry with me for the rest of my life, it's to raise an awareness of how incredibly alone and unsupported you feel as a mum-to-be when given the diagnosis. We made our decision not just for the best for us, but for the best for our family.

I/we were worried how such a big change would impact on our two-year-old's life. How we'd physically and mentally cope. Financially, how it would work. But above all else, we worried for the health of our unborn child. How many ops might they have to have, would we even make it to full-term – these are all things the NHS are very quick to remind you of. And for them, I genuinely believe (based on our experience) that it is black and white. They tell you how many people terminate after a result like ours and make you feel like it's the 'kindest' option. I know that while it would have been a huge shock, if we had never known, then we'd have loved, cherished and supported a baby with DS in the same way we would any baby. But whether I'd have had the strength and courage to do it as well as you clearly do, Sarah, I don't know and never will.

I hope me sending you this message has not upset or angered you. Like I say, I've held off for a long time in sending it. But please know that it comes from a place of wanting to share my experience and to help in raising awareness by supporting women, couples and entire families with the same diagnosis we had. Two months on to the day, and I still think about the decision we made, how it's changed our view on life and what you shouldn't take for granted. I hope you're able to be my voice on this, and share my message. As until they support and educate women like me in the right way, post a DS diagnosis, there will continue to be many missed opportunities to learn how much of a fulfilling life children born with DS can lead. And we'll continue to see less of them in our day to day lives. Thanks for your time Sarah.

With much respect.

Anon

CHAPTER EIGHTEEN

'Friends become our chosen family.'

'It's Oscar – hi, Oscar,' I heard a little voice shout over the noise of the preschool room. We'd just walked through the door and the boy who'd noticed us walk in came over and he and Oscar greeted each other with a big hug. It was a lovely exchange and made me smile.

I realised that I hadn't seen the little boy in the preschool room before and, considering his size, I thought he was probably just starting. He knew Oscar from when they used to be in the younger children's room. As I left them to it, I also noted that it had been a long while since Oscar had been greeted that way. I mean sure, he always gets a warm welcome from the staff but it dawned on me that the kids his own age, the kids all fast approaching school age, didn't seem that fussed by Oscar any more. Not like they used to be anyway.

And don't get me wrong, Oscar couldn't have cared less. He'd stroll in confidently, hang up his coat and bag on his peg (with my help, of course) and then off he'd go. He didn't seem fazed in the slightest that none of the other kids were in the least bit bothered by him being there. It was just me ... over-sensitive, over-protective me. Because here's the thing: while I knew Oscar had 'friends', I could also sense a shift in those friendships, as his mainstream-typical peers had started to grow up and Oscar, although doing well in so many areas, had in most areas lagged behind.

I always hear the phrase, 'Our kids are more alike than different.' This references the fact children with Down syndrome are much like their mainstream typical peers. I think this is true in a lot of ways. Oscar was cheeky just like most other (almost) four-year-olds. He was inquisitive, adventurous, caring and sensitive to how you're feeling. He was determined but defiant just as much as the next kid. But, in a lot of ways, he was, and still *is* to this day, very different from his typical peers. I'm not saying always, but sometimes he'd act differently to other kids. When he was upset or unsettled he'd chew on his fingers and cry. When he'd get excited, he'd run in circles doing his breathing in and out of his nose thing. When he'd get cross, he'd headbutt doors (seriously, I mean what is that about?). When his brother Alfie would fall over, instead of helping him up like other four-year-olds might, he'd drop to the floor dramatically himself. So, yeah, he didn't always behave the same way typical kids would but that's because he wasn't typical.

You see, I kinda felt, back then, that he was in this in-between stage. When he was younger, other kids his age had no idea he was any different to them, but now friends his age had become more aware and it was suddenly really obvious to me that they saw him differently. I will never forget the time that Oscar, a couple of his friends his age, and a nineteen-month-old were playing in the kitchen. The oven was on and, knowing a certain someone was not to be trusted, I walked in and told them that perhaps it'd be a good idea if we all went to play in the living room, instead. To which one of the little boys (Oscar's age) turned to me and said, 'Yes, the babies aren't allowed to play in here, either.' And just like that, I realised that he was referring not only to the nineteen-month-old but also to Oscar as one of those 'babies'. In his eyes, because Oscar was not able to talk to him like his other friends could, he was classed as a baby. Simple as that. And I got it. To an almost-four-year-old, when a child a little bit smaller than them in stature, is still in nappies and lacks the capability to engage in conversation, in their eyes, of course they're younger than them, even though they might be the same age.

Oscar and his friends would play together beautifully sometimes but other times, he might decide to tip the entire contents of the toy box onto the floor because he knew it'd make a great big noise that he liked. When this happened the other kids his age would look on in bewilderment. And when Oscar would decide that he'd like to join in the girls' roleplay game at nursery, when they would all lie in their makeshift bed, with their blankets over them, sometimes he would whip off all the blankets and run away with them, laughing to himself. I'd watch as this would unfold. Oscar now met with shouts of, '*Noo, Oscar!* Stop it. I was playing with that first.' And every once in a while, when Oscar would decide to give his friend a hug because, well, he quite fancied one, he'd go in for the tightest, longest hug imaginable, leaving said friend looking up at me with a 'Please save me' look in their eyes, because, well, it was kinda squishing them, I guess. You see, Oscar didn't always understand that tipping the contents of the toy box on the floor was just annoying. And stealing the girls' blankets? Yeah, so not cool. Oh, and the tight hug thing? Oscar hadn't quite grasped the whole personal space/boundaries thing. We as adults obviously get why Oscar does all of the above but for an almost-four-year-old, although they might like

Oscar and thought him fun at times, I think mostly they found him kind of annoying.

It wasn't just the four-year-olds though. Even Alfie, at two, had started looking at me slightly puzzled by some of the stuff Oscar would do. And quite honestly, I didn't blame any of them. I totally and utterly got why they'd react that way. Hey, when Oscar did some of the things he did, I myself raised an eyebrow, too.

But then there was one time we'd been in the park and some older kids, I presume around seven or eight, had taken a shine to Oscar. He stood there watching them play for a while, then started laughing at them because they were jumping off the climbing frame. The more Oscar laughed, the more they played up to him. The jumps became bigger. The pretend falls to the ground became more melodramatic. And the more Oscar dissolved into fits of giggles, the more attention they paid him. They helped him as he climbed up to join them and talked to him and even though he couldn't talk back, they didn't seem to mind. They accepted him just as he was, regardless, and as we moved away, I heard the two kids say to each other, 'Aah, he was so cool, wasn't he?'

'Yeah – so funny.'

My point being, when kids are a bit older, they might 'see' different, but they're OK with that. It was around this sort of time, just before Oscar was about to start school, that I wondered if and when the whole DS thing should be brought up with his peers. Initially, I thought it'd be much later down the line, but suddenly I was worrying perhaps it should be spoken about now. Some people might be of the opinion that nothing needs to be or should be said. Some think the sooner the better and others might say wait until they ask. There was a part of me that thought children Oscar's age are just these small people who couldn't possibly understand but then there was the other side of me, the side that hears a child refer to Oscar as 'naughty Oscar', that felt it might be best to sit them down there and then and explain that it's not that he's naughty, just that it takes him a little longer to understand.

On 21 March, World Down Syndrome Day, that particular year, a whole bunch of us were going round to a friend's house for lunch. My friends had suggested we all wear mismatched socks, including the kids, and as I arrived I was so incredibly touched that all of them, every single one, had remembered to put their brightly coloured socks on. I had wondered though, had the kids not questioned why they were being asked to put on odd socks that day? Did they not think it was ridiculous and want an explanation? I asked my friends. A couple said that their kids hadn't even noticed. Another said that she made a game out of it and said, 'I know, wouldn't it be really funny if we all wore different socks today?'

Which was met with a giggly 'OK'. But then there was one other. The little girl who – had I had to put money on it – would have been the one I said would be the kid who'd have questioned such silly antics. So when her mother said that they were to wear mismatched socks today, her response was, of course, 'Why, mummy?'

My friend had then told her daughter that it was World Down Syndrome Day and that they were going to wear them because Oscar and his family celebrate it. The little girl thought for a while and then asked, 'What's Down syndrome?' Her mummy, a very dear friend of mine, who was more than capable of explaining it to her little girl, told me that rather than launching into it there and then, she had deflected the question and asked me later that day what I would like her to say. What *did* I want her to say? What did I want any of my friends to say to their children? What did I think Chris and I would say to Alfie and Flo when they were old enough to understand a little more? What do they then say to their friends when they're asked the question, 'How come our brother looks, talks and acts that way?' At what point did I want them to say it? Today? Next month? Next year? In a couple of years? I wasn't sure. Some children, like the little girl who was puzzled by the mismatched socks, might have been ready for that chat but for others it may not have been the right time.

I guess I wanted the parents to say that Oscar was just a little boy. That, yes, he was a little different to them but that was OK. I wanted them to say that just because he acted the way he did at the moment, they must try not to get cross and try to be patient if they could. That things just take him a little longer to understand, but that he'd get there in the end. I'd like them to tell the children that Oscar may find some things harder than other people do but that perhaps there are some things they might find difficult in their lives, too. Not everyone's going to be good at everything, after all. What I know I would have loved them to tell them though, is all about Oscar's strengths. That he's brilliant on the trampoline and on his scooter. That he can run super-fast just like they can. Oh, and when they're feeling sad, Oscar will always notice and he'll give them the biggest hugs. But most importantly that just because he can't talk to them at the moment, it didn't mean he never would. One day, hopefully, he'd be able to tell them exactly what he's thinking and feeling.

I'm guessing my worries were heightened because later that year Oscar was starting school. I knew he'd be supported well, as thankfully we did get the one-to-one hours he needed in place, but I worried a lot about friendships forming. I know that in his own unique way he'd be able to communicate with his classmates but would they have the patience to persevere? All any mother wants for their child is for them to be liked. Of course, none of us can tell our children who to be friends with or who to like. They're going to make up their own minds, Even at the grand old age of four. All we can do is hope that they find their own way in life.

We can't tell our kids how to act, feel or who to like (and I would hate for other children to feel forced to be friends with Oscar) but I hope that one day, his peers will understand just what he's about. A little boy more like them than different, sure, but someone that they want to be around, regardless.

Blog comments

We have Purdy, who is soon to be four. Our diagnosis was postnatal and the world went from under our feet. I grieved and raged and thought unspeakable things. However, I laugh more now than ever I did before (and her two big sisters are funny), my love for Purdy has a thick layer of ferocious on top of it. You don't know the power you possess until you walk a path like this one. I have long since forgiven myself for those early feelings. I needed them back then. They inched me closer to acceptance. Do I wish I had known before? Yes, *but* only if I had been given balanced and reassuring information when I was told she had DS. Lessening the shock would, for me, have been better but would I change Purdy or our journey? Nope! I am neither religious nor patient and yet I am beyond happy at this unexpected twist in our tale.

Davina O'Donoghue

After some miscarriages, I went through very thorough studies and at a very early stage I was given the amazing news that I was pregnant with a girl but I should terminate her because it was almost certain she was coming with severe deformation and DS. That started my worst nightmare in my life and for the first time I was scared, but now at nine months Salma is proving me that I allowed others to take control of my feelings, I didn't gave her the opportunity to feel my unconditional love, I was just trying to protect her from everybody who was trying to convince me to terminate her. She's almost walking now, babbling 'Papa' and 'Mama'. No health issues, no deformations, just the extra chromosome 21 which from my perspective is just more love! As soon I felt her inside me, I wanted to give her the chance for life, she fought for that right herself!

Susana Arias De Reay

Hello, I have followed your blog for a while now and just wanted to write to say what a worthwhile and important job you are doing. When I was pregnant with my first son over five years ago we were told we had a 'high risk' pregnancy. Our baby's nuchal measurement was above what it should be and combined with blood tests we were told he had a high risk of Down syndrome. To be honest, the doctors put the fear of God into us; we had many scans and serious-faced doctors told us all the risks until we were very overwhelmed and pretty terrified of what it all meant. I knew I was having my baby regardless, but our only positive experience came from a wonderful midwife who pulled me and my husband into a side room after our meeting with the doctor, and told us that if our baby did indeed have Down syndrome there was a lot of support where we live and that our baby would have a happy and fulfilling life. I felt like she had thrown me a life raft. We opted for CVS testing (chorionic villus sampling), which was a massive ordeal, but I just wanted to know so I could prepare, really. So while waiting for the results I spent every waking hour on the internet researching what our future could hold and if I had come across your page back then I would have found it massively reassuring and it would have helped confirm my feelings that things would have actually been OK. It turned out our boy didn't have Down syndrome, but those weeks will stay with me for ever, as will the midwife's kind and sensible words. So, really, I just wanted to say, keep doing what you are doing – sharing your gorgeous family and being the life raft to other worried mums. Hope you don't mind me writing.

Jennifer Hayes

CHAPTER NINETEEN

'If you have something worth fighting for,
then fight for it.'

We were in the process of trying to finalise Oscar's EHCP. We had asked the local authority for the document to include his entitlement to a one-to-one key worker the entire time he was in school. We got that without a battle, but the OT and speech therapy was taking some time to finalise.

Our caseworker had sent us Oscar's draft EHCP and because we were not altogether happy with the provisions, we sent it back with our amendments (something you're allowed to do – not just us being cheeky). It seemed, though, that we weren't really getting any definitive answers back about any of it, so I asked my caseworker if I could exercise my right to a meeting with her and the therapists. In that meeting, the

OT said what they thought Oscar should be awarded therapy-wise and I said what I thought. Ultimately, as most things, the caseworker needed to go back to her manager to see if they'd come round to my way of thinking and honour what I was asking for. I told the caseworker that if we didn't get what we needed, we would take it to an appeal and tribunal. I also said that, by law, they now had to take into consideration the report written by Oscar's private occupational therapist, not just the NHS-employed OT who was at the meeting. While I understood there were financial limitations and that there were lots of children needing the service, I knew that they were not legally allowed to make a decision based on funding or budgets but solely on what was best for the child.

I asked the OT what she thought the chances were of her manager signing off my requests. She looked doubtful. 'To be honest with you,' she said, 'I've never known any child of Oscar's age be allocated as much as you're asking for.'

'OK,' I said, 'but have you ever met a mum on as much of mission like me before?'

'No,' she replied with a little laugh.

I told her that the Down syndrome community was a small one. That I was no different from any parent out there, simply trying to get what their child needs. I told her we were well aware of our rights and, really, all any of us wanted was what was best for our children. I had friends with children with DS who had gone through or were currently going through this EHCP process. They were supportive, encouraging and helped me along the way with it all. Without them, I'm not altogether sure I would have known how to go about any of it.

I don't think I'm the first parent and I'm sure I won't be the last to say that the thought of my child starting school filled me with mixed emotions. It seemed like five minutes ago he was a tiny baby in my arms and here we were, just a couple of months to go before he was due to start school and I couldn't believe it had come round so quickly. We were excited for him. We couldn't wait to see how he'd get on. And although I knew in my heart of hearts we had made the right decision in regard to seeing how he went in a mainstream school I still, of course, had my worries. It's a daunting time for any parent with a child starting school but for a child with additional needs and all the added worry that comes with it, I'm sure it's pretty normal to be apprehensive.

A few weeks later Chris and I had a transition meeting at Oscar's new school. Attending the meeting was one of Oscar's class teachers (who also happened to be the SENCo), his SENCo and key person from nursery, his physio, his PSS (the hearing impairment person), his early support key worker, the early years improvement advisor and his early support co-ordinator, who chaired the meeting. If I'm honest with you, I had felt a bit anxious. When I told them that I hadn't been successful toilet-training Oscar yet (and although I would endeavour to give it a go before he started, I knew he just wasn't there yet), they couldn't have been more brilliant about it. I was worried about telling them that, having stopped for a good while, that Oscar had reverted back to biting on occasion. Would that worry them? Would it put them off wanting him? My fear was unwarranted, for it didn't appear to faze them in the slightest.

I came away feeling like a weight had been lifted off my shoulders. They couldn't have been more supportive or more understanding, but what I gained most from the meeting was the knowledge that everyone there only had Oscar's best interests at heart. I think as parents we can sometimes focus on all the bad stuff, what our kids aren't achieving yet, and let that overshadow all the really positive things about them.

As we sat around the table and I listened to everything everyone was saying about Oscar – how much the nursery staff appeared to love him, how the professionals that worked with Oscar valued him and were proud of him – I had a feeling that everything would be OK.

I'm not sure if it was just me, perhaps it was, but as a parent with a child like Oscar going into a mainstream setting, I felt, rightly or wrongly, just that tiny bit grateful. Grateful that we had come so far. Grateful that kids like Oscar were accepted and actually wanted in a local school. I think before there would have been a part of me that worried whether Oscar actually would be wanted. We'd looked round other local mainstream schools and, although they didn't say they didn't want him, the subtext couldn't have been any more obvious that they didn't – I'm thinking of the school I described earlier whose SENCo had suggested I keep Oscar back a year. After that meeting with our chosen school, I felt a new-found confidence. It just reaffirmed for me that we were absolutely doing the right thing by him and that the school genuinely was looking forward to having him there.

The morning came for Oscar to have his first settling-in session at the school. As we approached the building, I started to explain to him that this was his new school and how exciting I thought it was (yep, over-enthusiastic mother alert!). All too quickly, though, I realised that Oz wasn't altogether fussed either way with the whole 'new school thing' and proceeded to shake his head, defiantly sit down in the middle of the school car park and refuse to move. Thankfully, there wasn't too much of a stand-off between the two of us as he saw a bunch of children playing in the playground, right next to the door we needed to go through and, thinking they looked like fun, he ran all the way to the entrance and through the door.

It was only then he realised there was a big crowd of people inside so he took a few tentative steps backwards, backing towards the door. A friendly teacher came over to greet us. She had a big warm smile and enthusiastically said, 'Hello,' but, realising Oz needed a bit of time, she gave us a bit of space for five minutes or so. I will admit, at this point, though, I was quite happy. Oscar, doing his 'I'm so shy, hiding behind my hands and looking out from behind them to check who's there' is obviously very endearing and it meant he wasn't charging in there like a bull in a china shop (the other side of Oscar that we frequently see which I'd earnestly hoped wouldn't come out that day).

This is going pretty well, I thought. Look how calm and collected he's being. I needn't have worried, he's even starting to play.

For the most part of the session, I was super-proud of him. He played for a long while in the kitchen, pretending to bake cakes, giving them out to all the parents and children. He even helped when one of the toy market stalls with all its fruit and veg got knocked over. He put them all back nicely.

This is going brilliantly, I thought.

Hmm.

I need to learn. To this day Oscar has a habit of lulling me into a false sense of security and then *bam*, ruins everything. And so it was that morning. The next thing I knew, he'd started emptying the box of dinosaur figures all over the floor. He ran to the sofa area, started flinging the soft toys off the sofa, at quite some speed I might add, missing his new classmates by an embarrassingly narrow margin, and then proceeded to lounge on the sofa, legs in the air, making himself quite at home.

'So how firm are you with him?' the teacher asked, watching him out of the corner of her eye. I knew why she was asking. She was trying to gauge how to approach it. Yes, he'd need more time to fully understand what's expected of him, she was probably thinking, but should he be allowed to get away with stuff just because he has Down syndrome?

I explained that usually I'm very firm, signing and saying a 'No' and always making him clear up the mess he's made.

She said, 'Good. That's good to know. Just so we can nip things in the bud from the start.'

As I left, I smiled to myself about her 'nipping it in the bud' comment. Yeah, good luck with that. I'd been trying to 'nip things in the bud' for the last four years now and it's still a work in progress.

The next settling-in session was scheduled for the Monday and, apparently, I was to leave him in their care and one of his key workers from nursery was going in to talk to his new teachers. I felt relieved I didn't have to attend. Don't get me wrong, I was sad he was growing up and it was massively pulling at the old heart strings watching him take this next big step. But not having to watch him cause trouble in the classroom? I think it was *much* better for my nerves that way. When I collected Oscar after the session, I watched as he came out the classroom, scanned the playground for me, saw me and then rushed over to me with the biggest, broadest grin, falling into my arms for the loveliest of hugs. Both the key worker from nursery and the teachers said he'd done brilliantly, exploring the different play stations and being well-behaved throughout the session. He sat on the floor and listened to a story at the end of his time. They then realised he'd rested his head on a nearby stool and had had a quick snooze. Obviously, he found it that exhilarating! The only time he got a little upset was when one of his friends, who he knows away from school, had started to cry and he'd reacted to him by crying a little, too. I thought if anything, that was really quite lovely, that he'd felt sad for his friend. I also met one of the TAs who would be looking after him next year. She'd been in the school a year, she told me, looking after another pupil with additional needs, but she used to be a teacher herself, before she'd taken a break to have her children.

We only live about a ten-minute walk from the school but it'd been playing on my mind: how was I going to do the school run with Oscar and the other two in the buggy? I knew he was more than capable of walking the distance but mindful that when he tires, he was likely to sit down in the middle of the path and not budge. Likewise, and probably more likely, was that he had a tendency to run ahead and had really no sense of danger whatsoever. I'd been worried about whether I'd be able to cope with him walking, while pushing the buggy. As Alfie was in nursery that day, I thought I'd give letting him walk to school a go. I took the double-buggy with me, Flo in one seat and the other spare in case Oscar tired. He coped brilliantly, walking all the way there and all the way back with no problems at all. He'd held my hand when I asked him to while crossing roads and didn't once run off.

A few days later I picked Oscar up from nursery to find him with a thin residue of black paint all over his face, in his ears and up his nostrils. The reason for said coverage was that Oscar had decided to paint his new shoes, his body, the corridor out to the nursery garden and part of the nursery garden wall. Having seen Oscar from afar covered in paint and then wandering around the corner to see a member of staff on the floor, bucket beside her, scrubbing the walls, it didn't take a detective to work out the series of events that had played out that afternoon after tea. And while the nursery staff couldn't have been lovelier (having told him off as soon as it had happened, they were telling me how funny they actually thought it was), I found myself despairing.

You see, we were having one of those weeks. In fact, we'd been having one of those weeks for a few months now! I'd been watching him like a hawk, just in case he'd get himself into trouble. I'd always remembered having a conversation with Hayley from Downs Side Up, who told me that she believed that the first year Natty was at school was the hardest. She said that while she was capable of so much, she still didn't quite 'get it yet' – and that was exactly how I felt about Oz at the moment. I knew I needed to chill out and realised that although it might all get worse before it gets better, you didn't see twenty-five-year-old grown men with Down syndrome charging around, painting walls black, do you? Oh god … *do* you?

The EHCP process was supposed to take twenty weeks and be based on the child's needs. After thirty-five weeks our report was completed and, totally ignoring our views as Oscar's parents and that of his private therapists, Oscar's EHCP was based on what the local authority wanted to pay for. They'd told me that if I disagreed I could take them to court. So that's what I did. My friend Karen summed up the process perfectly. She said, 'Raising a child with additional needs is easy but the paperwork the government put you through to access the things they are entitled to is time-consuming, emotionally stressful, frustrating and a total inefficient use of resource and tax payers' money.'

Oscar hadn't started school yet but he was literally just about to. We got the tribunal court date through for a few months after his start date, 3 January 2017 (Happy New Year to me) and until then we would have to sit and wait. It was, however, just so very frustrating that what it ultimately came down to was that the local authority were constrained by diminishing budgets and reduced resources. It's a joke the lengths families have to go to get what their children need and deserve. I didn't think I had ever felt the complete injustice of the system so strongly before. Ever.

The day that he was to begin school finally came. I remember feeling sick to my stomach. All morning (he didn't go in until after lunch as his school did staggered starts), I had a lump in my throat and was on the brink of tears. How had we got here? We'd come so far. Thinking back to his birth, his diagnosis and all that followed. It had been a living nightmare. But now look at us. Here he was, about to start mainstream school.

One of the things I found hardest to come to terms with was the fact that Oscar couldn't articulate to me, his TAs or teachers how he'd be feeling. Sure, if he was upset or unwell, I knew him well enough to recognise the signs. But if he became unhappy in school, he wouldn't be able to tell me just yet. He couldn't tell me if someone was nasty to him or if he'd had a bad day and equally and just as sad for me, he wouldn't be able tell me if he loved his new school and all about any new friends he might have made. By the same token, when I think about the diagnosis of Down syndrome we got after he was born and what we thought it meant for him, I never for one moment dreamt he'd be the little boy he'd become by that day. I was excited to see what the future held for him and so incredibly proud of how far our boy had come.

When he walked in, although he looked a little nervous at the change, he didn't even glance back. And the expression on his face when he ran out to greet me after he'd finished for the day said it all. Although, at first, Oscar only started doing a few hours at a time, he did so well. Every morning, he managed to walk to school with no problems. He walked along beside me and I thought it was interesting to see that when he saw other children holding their mummy's hands, he'd wanted to hold mine, too. Something he'd never normally instigate. Towards the end of his first week, however, he'd stepped out the front door and signed that he wanted to get in the car and got a little tearful when I said we had to walk. Thankfully, he got to ride on the front step of the buggy I was pushing Alfie and Flo in, so no problem there and he perked up by the time we got to school. If on day one and two, he'd walked in looking pretty apprehensive, by week two he was walking in without a care in the world, and didn't seem fazed at all. The school started a communication diary that the TAs, teachers and I could write in, sharing information on a day-to-day basis. We wrote how the day had gone or any information I had about what sort of weekend or night he'd had.

So all in all, I'd say it was a success. The fact that one morning shortly after he started, he went and got his uniform and shoes to change into, without me even mentioning school, was encouraging, and when we drove past the school he pointed and shouted, '*Mum, mum, mum – yeeeahh!*' There were only three other places that prompted a cheer when we drove past or arrived at them – the park, his grandparents' house or an ice-cream van. I think I can be fairly confident in saying that school got the big thumbs-up from Oscar.

Blog comments

Hi Sarah. I don't know how I came across you on Facebook/Instagram but I'm so glad I did. I am a parent of two grown-up kids (twenty and eighteen). Neither of them has additional needs, not that this has anything to do with anything really! I know so much about you I thought

I would share something about me. What I
wanted to tell you was that *you* make me smile
and laugh out loud almost every day. I love your
honesty about parenting, your challenges and
your achievements. Your facial expressions are
fantastic, you don't need to say a word!

Clare Murphy

CHAPTER TWENTY

'*A correct diagnosis is three-fourths the remedy.*'
– Mahatma Gandhi

We were at an appointment with the paediatrician, who suggested that in another year we might like to do an assessment on Oscar to see if he had ADD (attention deficit disorder). I could say it was a shock, except she was the third professional in the space of a few months who had uttered that three-letter acronym. Three letters that cut a little deeper every time they were mentioned.

The paediatrician's office was sparse. Lots of space, a bed, a few chairs, a device for measuring your height and a chair to sit on to measure your weight. As the doctor and I discussed Oscar's progress and any medical issues that arose in the last six months, Oscar jumped up on to the bed, standing on a conveniently placed box to heave himself up. It wasn't done with any sort of grace or decorum. More like a bull in a china shop. He sat there for a while, jumped off, and started playing with the height measure, clumsily knocking it over as he moved on. He flitted from one chair to another and, if I'm completely honest with you, he wasn't still for much longer than a few seconds at a time.

'It's not something we'd be thinking about yet,' the paediatrician said of the ADD assessment, 'more so when he's around five or six years old. He's still so young, it could be that it's an immaturity thing. There's not that much in this room to keep him occupied. But I'm noticing today, nothing's really holding his attention. What do you think, Mrs Roberts?'

She was right. I knew she was right. He wasn't sitting still at all and if I was her, I'd totally think he had ADD. And to tell you the truth, it had been something I'd been thinking about for a long while now. But equally, I genuinely had thought that in the last few months he had calmed down. He seemed to be playing with toys at home more than he ever did before. He now enjoyed sitting and listening to a story being read to him (he would never have done that six months ago). He never used to sit and watch TV, but would invariably be doing some sort of acrobatics off the sofa. And that had definitely stopped. So what I thought, truthfully, was that he'd calmed down considerably and that meant the niggling thought at the back of my mind about ADD might have been wrong.

I told the paediatrician she wasn't the first to raise the suggestion. His thyroid consultant had asked me about his attention a month or so earlier, when he'd climbed on the bed in her surgery and intermittently played with the curtains. His OT attributed his energy levels to his sensory-seeking and said that if we could find ways to manage that, she was certain he'd calm down. But who knew who was right here?

What I do know is that day in the paediatrician's room, my heart hurt again. It didn't hurt the way it did when I got the potential Down syndrome diagnosis. That was another level of pain. But it hurt at the thought of Oscar having yet another diagnosis marked against his name. I felt cross that this kid had enough to deal with in the four short years he'd been on this planet. He didn't need another label, surely? The paediatrician reassured me that it may not be the case at all and that it might just be that he was young and being a 'typical' boy. But she said that we needed to be on top of it from an educational/ learning point of view if it turned out he did indeed have ADD. She said before our next appointment she would ask the school for a report from their perspective. She'd ask how his focus and attention was, how he was learning, how he was getting on generally. Listening to her I thought that the other kids I've been around who have DS were probably not as lively as Oscar. Maybe my deep-rooted fears were about to be confirmed?

I guess what I'm most gutted about was my reaction. I'm going to be honest. I have always vowed I would be honest here. I was cross with myself because I did exactly the same as I had when I found out Oscar had DS. I panicked, imagining all the things that that label meant, without really knowing much about it. I had an idea in my mind of what having a child with DS meant and could only think of that. The reality, I later found out, of course, was far removed. But I was now doing the same thing with ADD. In my head, all I could think of when I thought of a child having ADD was them charging around, out of control and unmanageable. I thought about despairing, frazzled parents, trying desperately to control their child but to no avail. I had the label in my mind, a fear about what ADD meant, before I'd even understood it and what it'd means for Oscar, and for that I was annoyed at myself.

The paediatrician concluded that *if* Oscar did have ADD, it could be managed with medication. I of course knew that and did feel some relief that there would be help out there, should he need it. If his focus and attention was better, surely that'd mean his learning would progress? That could only be a positive. But I felt sad that day because I realised this could potentially mean, *more* medicine. *More* intervention. *More* challenges.

I knew that whatever happened, there was no point in worrying about it now. A lot can change in six months to a year and it didn't sound as though the paediatrician was going to be assessing him anytime soon. It didn't change anything really, he was still my gorgeous little boy and if he happened to have ADD, too, we would tackle it head-on, as we always tried to do. The thing I've realised is that life has a habit of throwing us these curveballs from time to time. It wouldn't change Oscar as a person at all. He was loved and that was all that mattered, ultimately. But perhaps I thought it'd change me again. Despite priding myself on trying to look on the brighter side of life and at the bigger picture (there are worse things that can happen in the world, right?) it felt like yet another setback, another grey hair or wrinkle (to add to the rest) and another dent in my already bruised heart.

They say that when you have a child, you become their biggest and fiercest protector. They also say the hardest part of being a parent is watching your child go through something really tough and not being able to fix it. I think 'they', whoever they are, have a point. The previous year, if Chris or I had been at a party with Oscar, if I'm honest with you, we would have been on high alert. He had a habit of trashing other people's houses. Not in a malicious way, but just because it was fun. Laundry baskets would be thrown downstairs with the entire contents of the basket on the hallway floor, plants would be de-potted, leaving a trail of soil behind him. In fact, wherever he went he'd often leave a trail of destruction. And then of course there was the biting. It had started when he was two, stopped for a bit, then started again for a while. We knew that it was more than likely down to his frustrations in communication, so that was another reason for Chris and I to shadow him the whole time at a party, just in case we needed to step in. It was exhausting, draining and we felt like we never spent any time talking to anyone else at these gatherings. We felt rude continuously saying, 'Excuse me, I've just got to check on Oz,' but it had to be done because more than anything we didn't want to be those parents that just stood there, unfazed by what their child was getting up to.

A year had made a big difference. After we had taken Oz to two parties, Chris and I commented that he'd come a long way. Now we didn't feel like we needed to watch him the whole time. He didn't destroy houses. He tried to play with the other kids. He was happy. He was engaged and he was no trouble at all. So why, if he was so much better than a year ago, did I go to bed after the first party, feeling just ever so slightly deflated? I think it's the 'party' thing. It really highlighted that sometimes, in a party or play situation, Oscar really does struggle sometimes. I've heard other parents of kids with additional needs also mention similar issues, although I'm not for a second speaking on behalf of every parent here as I know that there's a lot of kids with additional needs who do brilliantly, who have lots of friends and wouldn't struggle at all socially.

Take for instance the first party this year. All the boys were charging up and down the garden and hiding behind the shed. Oscar was joining in, just about able to keep up, but I saw that his little brother Alfie was seemingly the ringleader at one point, running ahead, shouting instructions to all the other kids, engaging in conversation with all of them. I realised that Oscar was silent. He was trying to engage. He was trying to get their attention. But I guess to the other four- and five-year-old boys, Oscar's idiosyncrasies (like the way he stands really close to you to get your attention or hits you on the back in a playful way as he runs past so you'll look at him) were just a bit odd. I watched as Oscar got a little too close to one of the boys and ended up bumping into him. Then I watched as this little boy turned around, looked him straight in the eye and said, 'I don't want to play with you', and ran off.

A year ago, Oscar wouldn't have given this a second thought and would have more than likely gone after him anyway. But this particular day Oscar stood there, his face dropped and his whole demeanour changed as he shrunk just a couple of inches. He had understood every word of 'I don't want to play with you'. He'd taken it all in and it had hurt.

Chris, aware of what was happening too, headed straight over to Oscar and, instead of making it into a big issue, encouraged Oscar to run with him and to catch up with the rest of the group, which obviously immediately lifted Oscar's mood. He had a great time after that, and the little boy's comment was probably the furthest thing from his mind as he enjoyed the rest of the party. But it had stayed with me.

Chris and I talked that night about the fact that we're really aware of how it is for Oscar in those situations. How other kids can be. That it must be really confusing for a four-year-old child to fathom out why Oscar acts the way he does and why he can't always answer when spoken to. It must be just as frustrating for them as it is for Oscar, I suppose.

But sometimes I really wish that little kids weren't so horrible.

At another party the other day, a little girl, exactly the same age as Oscar, asked me how old he was. We'd just had a brief conversation about the fact that Oscar could only say a few words at the moment but that hopefully someday he'd be able to talk like her. It had come up because Oscar had bumped into her (yep, this boy is clumsy) and hadn't said 'Sorry' and she came to tell me what had happened. I explained that it was an accident, that he definitely would have been sorry, just that he couldn't actually say the word 'sorry' yet (as an aside, he can sign 'sorry' but more than likely decided not to, knowing him). She'd taken it all on board and that was when she asked his age.

'He's four,' I said. She looked at me, puzzled.

'Yes, but he's only just four because I'm nearly five,' she said, because in her mind, I guess, if he were nearly five and her age, then of course he'd be able to talk.

'Well,' I explained, 'he's four at the moment and he was born the same month you were.'

And with that, thinking about it for a second or two, off she went.

As a parent, it's hard to watch the kids not having the tolerance or patience with him. Don't get me wrong, I totally understand the reasons, but it's still hard. He tries so hard to engage and can do so in many ways – it's just that the words aren't there yet and for other four-year-olds, that's just weird, right?

So, as a parent of the child who can't fight back, when do you step in and say something?

I'm the parent in the park, who is always standing next to the play equipment where my kids are playing because they're either all too young to be left alone or, in Oscar's case, too vulnerable to be without support. I'm definitely not the parent sat on the park bench outside the children's play area, out of eyesight, chilling out with my coffee and talking to a friend. So I hear everything. I hear how kids are with one another. And I know for a fact that it's not only children like Oscar who are told they don't want to be played with. Kids are blatant. They say it how it is. They talk about who are their friends and who aren't. Who their *best* friends are – a classic at that age. The sad thing is, this isn't a new thing because I remember as a child doing exactly the same thing. But with all that in mind, I'm also the parent in the park who will step in. Whether the child is Oscar or not. If another child is being horrible and their parents aren't around, I'll call them up on it. Because, well, they need to be told, right?

I said there were two parties that we took Oscar to and noticed the change in him and, interestingly, the second party was different for me as well. They had an entertainer who was fabulous but fairly loud and for the first part of the party a dubious Oscar stayed close to me. But ever so slowly, as his confidence grew, we edged closer to the entertainer, where all the other kids were, and although it took him a while, he got involved in the end. And when I watched really closely (because now in a party situation, I can actually sit and have a chat with other mums because Oscar doesn't need me as much as he once did), he danced with some of the other kids, played with a balloon with another little boy and at the end, when the entertainer asked all the kids to huddle together for a photograph with the birthday boy, I watched as Oscar put his arm round a little girl and held the hand of the boy next to him. The girl and boy didn't think anything of it and gave him big smiles. As we left the party, it dawned on me that as long as he's having fun and feeling involved, that was all that mattered. The experience reaffirmed for me the fact that sometimes communication isn't about what you can say. It taught me Oscar can engage without saying anything at all and despite his efforts to say more (and we're getting more sounds all the time), perhaps for now Oscar doesn't need words.

Aside from the lack of speech, one of my biggest worries for Oscar has always been that he won't make friends. I worry he won't fit in. People talk about how society is changing and how we're all so much more accepting, especially the younger generation, but sometimes I'm not convinced. Oscar was due to go back to school after the two-week break for Easter and the evening before I busied myself, sorting out his PE kit and packing his bag. His communication book was in there, the document that went back and forth between home and his TA. It covered everything that either side might need to know and it was really lovely for Chris and I to hear how he'd gotten on each day, but as I reached for it that night, something fell out the bottom. It was a note and a drawing from a child in Oscar's class. This little boy had drawn a picture for Oscar and on the back had written 'Oscar' with a love heart and his name. It made me smile. Not because it was a big deal. But sometimes these little things, in their simplicity, are sent to us at exactly the right time we need them.

Blog comments

Hi, Sarah, I have loved your blog and updates, not as a person who has been personally affected by Down syndrome or as a mum of a special needs child, but just as a mum who wants her children to grow up with compassion, understanding and a desire to make people feel valued and welcome whatever their position/disability in life. I've talked to my kids often about the need to be inclusive, often with anecdotes from your blog. And today I discovered they had been listening to me after all! My twelve-year-old daughter came home from school and said a boy with DS had come and sat next to her at break at school, while she was talking with her friends. She'd never met him before and assumed he had just started year seven. He held her hand and wouldn't let go. This encroachment of her personal space by a boy (any boy for that matter) in front of her teenage friends was no doubt a little unsettling. But she turned to

him and asked him how his day was going, was he
enjoying school and what lesson did he have next
and could he find the way there all right. When the
bell to signal the end of break went and she got
up to leave, he got up, too, and held her hand the
whole way out. I was so proud of her when she
recounted the incident at the end of the day – for
her understanding that all people are different,
that she included him in her conversation with her
friends and that she made him feel comfortable,
even if it was bit unsettling for her at first. And
that's in large part because the messages you put
out there make us all think as parents and to have
that conversation with our children. And today, it
paid off for one child, in one instance. But every
little helps, right? Thank you.

Kate

CHAPTER TWENTY-ONE

*'I am proud of many things in my life but nothing
beats being a mother.'*

Who'd have thought we'd have made it here?
There I'd been, that rabbit stuck in the headlights, looking to Chris to tell me that it'd all be OK,
but he couldn't have possibly have seen this. He couldn't
have seen how our life would have panned out.

Oscar's settled well into school, with both Alfie and
Flo following behind him. Before we know it, they'll
all be together in the same school, which is something I
could only have dreamed of, way back when. And you
know what? Life is actually pretty good. Aside from the
odd hurdle along the way, which I'm getting pretty good
at negotiating, we're all leading happy and full lives.

I'd worried about so much in the beginning – how

having him would affect the family dynamic. Would we be able to cope? But the truth is we do, not just because we want to but because we have to.

I really hope that people don't feel sorry for us. I hope they see a family, just like any other, navigating their way through life, trying desperately hard to figure it all out, one day at a time. I hope they see that we're not all that different to the next family, really, just with some added extras.

I had a conversation with a friend whose child has Down syndrome. Coincidently, both of us have gone on to have another child (or in my case two) afterwards. Alfie and Flo and my friend's second child are all, as far as we are aware, 'typically developing' (I mean I would say 'normal' but first, that's clearly not very PC and second, what is normal anyway?). We talked about life, work, kids, etc., but then the subject turned (as it often does when you have something in common) to Down syndrome. My friend said to me that after having her second child, it took her a long while to adjust and to figure out that to her littlest one, she was simply just a mum. For so long with her first, yes, she'd of course been her mum, but she'd also been her teacher, her speech therapist, her occupational therapist, her physio. Her first had depended on her so much, for so long. She'd realised that the Down syndrome and all that came with the diagnosis (the appointments, the input these kids need) had taken over. But with her second – she really only needed to be her mum.

As we talked more, we both said that since having our other children, we've realised how much harder work the first children have been from the point of view that there is extra worry, extra appointments and extra energy required. We commented how much simpler life is with the others. And that's no disrespect to the older ones who happen to have DS, for obviously we love them. But it's the truth. We noted that with our younger ones there have been behavioural phases, but they've been short-lived. For example, all our younger ones now are far surpassing their older siblings in their language development. We realised that it was actually OK to admit all this stuff out loud to one another because – between us – there would be no judgement. I spoke openly about the fact that sometimes it made me sad to admit that things don't come as easily to Oscar as they do to my other two; seeing him struggle hurts. When he wakes in the night and I go to him for the twenty-hundredth time to resettle him, I admitted that sometimes I lose my patience.

When he woke up the other morning, having done a big old poop in his nappy that had literally gone everywhere (up his back, down his legs, all over the sheets), I told her I'd cursed under my breath and felt hard done by because I was sure other mums of children his age wouldn't have to be dealing with this still. When he sits or lies down on the floor because he's too tired to walk any further, I confessed to feeling exasperated having to carry him home on my shoulders, because he's so heavy now. Sometimes he goes into the kitchen cupboard and pours the sugar over the floor for no apparent reason, other than it is actually pretty fun, and I readily admitted I felt frustrated. When another child calls him naughty, I told her it cuts deep because all I want them to do is understand that he's not and that he's really just trying to figure it all out.

The battles for his EHCP, the surgeries, his diagnosis – sometimes I look at other people around me and feel envious that they don't have to deal with this themselves. I admit that sometimes Chris and I have neglected our relationship because of all of the above, because it can at times become all-consuming and our focus has had to be on Oscar (although this may just be having too many kids in close succession). And although in many ways Oscar is simpler than the other two, at least I can reason with them, because they understand consequences just that little bit more. Parenting the two of them is easier.

Yes, I've learnt more about patience and understanding and strength and resilience and the importance of having a thick skin and the fire in my belly to fight for everything he wants and deserves over the years. And yes, I truly love him with my full heart, but sometimes it'd be really lovely not to have to worry about any of the above and just simply be his mum. The thing is that over the years, I have realised that life has a habit of finding a way of keeping you on track, even when you hit a bumpy bit, we just keep on keeping on, right?

Chris once said something that has always stayed with me: 'When you're having a bad day, whether it's something at work, something to do with the kids, whatever, Oscar doesn't necessarily say anything, but he gives you this look that lets you know everything's going to be OK, doesn't he?' It looks so stupid, writing that, but I knew exactly what Chris meant. Oscar really does do that.

I'm not religious. I'm not even sure what I believe in at all these days. But what I do know is that Oscar is here to teach us what life is really about and, do you know what? I couldn't be more thankful.

And if you ask me what I would have liked to have known, to have told you, on the day Oscar was born and his DS diagnosis felt as if it had shattered our world – it would be to tell you that everything would turn out just fine.

I'd tell you that Oscar would do well and that all those worries in the beginning were pointless, really. Yes, some things have taken him longer to grasp but in some areas he's doing brilliantly and I have every faith that he'll get there in the end. I'd tell you that he loves school, has formed friendships amongst his peers. That he annoys his brother and sister in the same way they annoy him, just as I'd always pictured they would, before the DS featured.

I'd let you know that Oscar is so loved. Not just by myself, Chris and his siblings but by our entire family, friends and I guess all the people who continue to follow our story. We go on holiday, I work – in fact, his diagnosis has opened up opportunities for me that I could never have dreamed of – and my life isn't the one of loss and regret that I feared it would be. Far from it. I haven't lost friends because my son happens to have Down syndrome, I've gained a bunch more.

I'm conscious of the future, what it might hold for Oscar and how he'll cope. Looking very far ahead at the moment is, if I'm honest, a scary prospect. But my hopes and aspirations for Oscar are much the same as those I have for my other two – that he continues to feel loved, that he feels valued and has self-worth and, above all, that he's happy. That's surely all any mother wants for her child.

ACKNOWLEDGEMENTS

To Oscar, without whom this book wouldn't have been possible.

To Alfie and Flo, who continue to provide me with an abundance of material if ever I'm approached to write Book No. 2. You guys think parenting a child with additional needs is hard? These two run me ragged (I love them dearly though)!

Chris, my husband, who I adore more than anything in the world but who keeps me grounded, claiming he only read the first of my blog posts because the rest are 'really long' and it would take him ages to read – and besides he's 'living it', so knows how the story goes.

My mum – *the* best mum I could have ever wished for (and for her childcare).

My dad – the man who knows when I need a new winter coat and still tells me to 'Mind how you go' when I drive on the motorway.

My sisters – my best friends.

Twiz – my person.

Extended family and friends – too many to mention, but I love you all.

My readers/followers – you guys rock. Never underestimate how your words of support lift me up, daily. I'm grateful to each and every one of you.

To anyone who has ever felt sorry – I hope you see now, there's no need.